PROFESSOR JENNIE BRAND-MILLER'S
LowGI DIET
for Gluten-free Cooking

OTHER TITLES IN THE **LOWGI**DIET SERIES

Low GI Essentials
Low GI Diet Handbook
Low GI Diet: Shopper's Guide 2012

Cookbooks
The Low GI Diet Cookbook
The Low GI Family Cookbook
The Low GI Vegetarian Cookbook

Specific Health Concerns:
Diabetes
Low GI Diet: Diabetes Handbook
Low GI Diet for Childhood Diabetes

PCOS
Low GI Diet for Polycystic Ovarian Syndrome

Weight-loss
Low GI Diet 12-week Weight-loss Plan

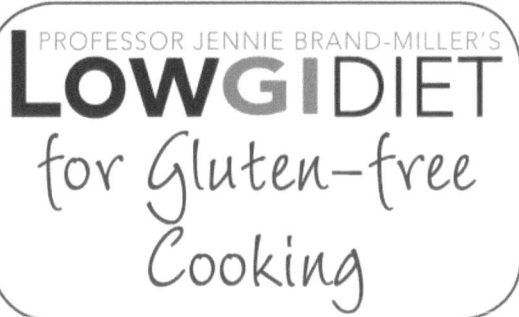

PROFESSOR JENNIE BRAND-MILLER'S
Low GI Diet for Gluten-free Cooking

Your Definitive Guide to
Using the Glycemic Index
for Gluten-free Living

**Prof Jennie Brand-Miller • Dr Kate Marsh
• Philippa Sandall**

With a foreword by Sue Shepherd,
Advanced Accredited Practising Dietitian

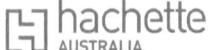

IMPORTANT NOTE TO READERS: Although every effort has been made to ensure that the contents of this book are accurate, it must not be treated as a substitute for qualified medical advice; always consult a qualified medical practitioner. Neither the authors nor the publisher can be held responsible for any loss or claim arising out of the use, or misuse, of the suggestions made or the failure to take medical advice.

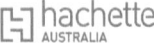

First published in Australia and New Zealand in 2007
by Hachette Australia (An imprint of Hachette Australia Pty Limited)
Level 17, 207 Kent Street, Sydney NSW 2000
www.hachette.com.au

Reprinted 2008, 2009
Revised 2010
This revised edition published in 2012

Text copyright © Dr Kate Marsh, Prof Jennie Brand-Miller, Philippa Sandall 2007, 2010, 2012

This book is copyright. Apart from any fair dealing for the purposes of private study, research, criticism or review permitted under the *Copyright Act 1968*, no part may be stored or reproduced by any process without prior written permission. Enquiries should be made to the publisher.

National Library of Australia Cataloging-in-Publication data:

Brand Miller, Jennie, 1952-
Low GI diet for gluten-free cooking / Jennie Brand-Miller, Kate Marsh, Philippa Sandall.
ISBN: 978 0 7336 2756 9 (pbk.)
Low GI diet series.
Includes index.
Cooking.
Gluten-free diet – Recipes.
Other Authors/Contributors:
   Marsh, Kate.
   Sandall, Philippa.
641.5638

Cover design by Judi Rowe, Agave Creative Group
Cover images courtesy of Shutterstock Images
Author photograph © Gavin Jowitt
Recipe testing and development by Diane Temple
Spice and herb blend recipes on pages 199 courtesy of Ian Hemphill, Herbie's Spices
Original text design by Pindar NZ, Auckland, New Zealand
Text design adaptation and typesetting by Kirby Jones

Contents

Foreword — vii
Introduction — 1

Part 1: *Going gluten-free* — 5
  1 Who really needs a gluten-free diet and why — 7
  2 Gluten-free ground rules — 15
  3 Gluten-free and low GI – why it matters — 23
  4 Your low GI, gluten-free food finder — 37

Part 2: *How do you do it* — 45
  5 Going gluten-free and low GI — 47
  6 Putting the GI to work in your day — 77

Part 3: *Eat yourself healthy* — 87
  7 Breakfasts and brunches — 95
  8 Snacks and treats — 111
  9 Light meals and lunches — 123
  10 Salads and soups — 141
  11 Mains — 159
  12 Desserts — 181
  13 Basics — 195

The GI gluten-free tables — 201
Contacts — 245
Acknowledgements — 249
About the authors — 250
Index — 252
Index of recipes — 258

Foreword

When I was first told the great news that this book was going to be written, I was thrilled. As a dietitian working in the area of coeliac disease for a very long time, I have seen first-hand the struggle many have faced in making their gluten-free diet varied, nutritious and enjoyable. As more and more people are aware of the importance of GI, combining this with the gluten-free diet has created some confusion about what to buy, what to cook and how to cook it! The *Low GI Diet for Gluten-free Cooking* really does take away such uncertainties and difficulties – it is packed full of ideas of how to accomplish a great-tasting gluten-free low GI diet.

There is no better team to write this enjoyable, informative book with delicious recipes. Kate Marsh, a well-respected dietitian, has both coeliac disease and diabetes herself. She has joined forces with Jennie Brand-Miller – noted worldwide for her ground-breaking research involving the glycemic index – and Philippa Sandall, who has a unique vision for great publications.

The *Low GI Diet for Gluten-free Cooking* is a book for many. It is ideal for people requiring both a gluten-free diet and a diet to assist with diabetes, heart disease, goals of weight or insulin control, and it appetisingly invites all people to incorporate low GI cooking into their lifestyle.

But it is more than just a recipe book. I commend the authors for a marvellous job in compiling useful information for readers, including background to the gluten-free diet, glycemic index and principles of healthy eating. The menu plans are so helpful. The comprehensive low GI gluten-free food list at the back of the book is an invaluable resource. The information and recipes have been compiled with such careful attention to detail – this is a great reference book of all things low GI and gluten-free.

I began taste-testing the recipes myself with the Barbecued Lemon Chicken Skewers and very soon after cooked the Pumpkin, Ricotta and Lentil Lasagne, and of course dessert! I could not turn the page past the Chocolate Almond Cake. My tastebuds were happy and content – but it was hard to resist going back for more. I am sure you, as readers of the delicious recipes contained within, will whole-heartedly agree.

I hope you enjoy this as much as I have.

Dr Sue Shepherd
Advanced Accredited Practising Dietitian
www.coeliac.com.au

Introduction

Having lived with type 1 diabetes since I was 10, and coeliac disease for the past few years, I've experienced first-hand the difficulties of following a restricted diet. And as a dietitian working with many people with the same conditions, I am only too well aware of the challenges faced by anyone trying to eat gluten-free, let alone trying to manage their blood glucose levels.

In fact, in my work, I have found that many adults and children with coeliac disease, in their attempt to follow a strict gluten-free diet, don't end up eating a particularly well-balanced diet.

And while for most people, the improvement in how they feel makes it easy to stick with their diet, I have also seen the struggle some have with:

- The lack of variety in their diet
- Feeling hungry all the time, and
- Running out of energy during the day.

That is why I have teamed up with Jennie and Philippa to write this book.

Gluten-free or not, eating well is the key to our health and wellbeing, so it pays to get it right.

The *Low GI Diet for Gluten-free Cooking* is for anyone with coeliac disease or a gluten intolerance who wants to maximise their health and energy levels by eating well. If you want to ensure that you still get all the nutrients your body needs, feel satisfied after meals, enjoy a varied diet despite restrictions and optimise your long-term health and wellbeing, then this book is for you.

WHY THIS BOOK IS IMPORTANT

There is much more to a gluten-free lifestyle than focusing on foods to avoid. Eating well is the key to good health for everyone, and eating the right foods gives the body the fuel it needs to perform at its best and the energy to get through the day. It's also an important part of managing and preventing other long-term health problems, including diabetes, heart disease, cancer and a range of digestive complaints.

While it is great to see an ever-increasing range of gluten-free foods becoming available and making life easier for those with coeliac disease, unfortunately many of them are highly processed and some are high in fat and added sugar – two ingredients that are naturally gluten-free!

Gluten-free diets also tend to have a high glycemic index (GI) – we explain what this is and why it matters in detail in Chapter 3. Many low GI staples such as whole wheat kernel breads, pasta, barley and oats are eliminated because they contain gluten. The gluten-free alternatives, due to their ingredients and processing methods, are often quickly digested and absorbed, raising blood glucose and insulin levels and leaving you feeling hungry and often low on energy a few hours after eating.

What this means in practice is that many people following a gluten-free diet are rarely satisfied after meals and may feel hungry between meals, which can lead to overeating and weight gain. As far as we know, this is the first book that shows you how to incorporate low GI carbs into your meals and reap their health benefits; including a reduced risk of pre-diabetes, type 2 diabetes, cardiovascular disease and some types of cancer. A low GI diet can also help diabetes sufferers manage their blood glucose levels. Since coeliac disease is more common in people with type 1 diabetes, this is particularly important. Low GI eating is for everybody, every day, every meal.

It can be difficult to get the right balance on a gluten-free diet, but it is certainly not impossible. In fact, we will show you just how easy it is in this comprehensive guide to what you should be eating, the things you need to leave out, and a fantastic selection of delicious recipes to tempt your tastebuds.

Dr Kate Marsh
Sydney

Once again, the team behind the Low GI Diet phenomenon have pulled together to bring you cutting-edge science and practical know-how to make a healthier, happier you. We are delighted to have Kate on board again (she helped us write the *Low GI Diet for Polycystic Ovarian Syndrome* and *The Low GI Vegetarian Cookbook*), who brings both her personal and professional experience of living and breathing a gluten-free diet. If you'd like to keep up-to-date with the latest GI science and GI values, subscribe to our free newsletter, *GI News*, at http://ginews.blogspot.com.

Prof Jennie Brand-Miller
and Philippa Sandall
Sydney

Part 1

Going gluten-free

For many adults and children, gluten-free eating is a lifesaver. But if it's not well planned, the result can be an unbalanced, unhealthy diet low in wholegrains and fibre and high in the fat and added sugar found in many of the gluten-free foods on supermarket shelves. And it is probably a high GI diet too, because slowly digested staples such as grainy breads, pasta, muesli and traditional porridge oats are off the menu.

Chapter 1 | Who really needs a gluten-free diet and why

Some people can't tolerate gluten. If you have coeliac disease or dermatitis herpetiformis (a gluten-sensitive chronic skin condition) you need to eat a gluten-free diet. For life. If you have a gluten intolerance (non-coeliac gluten sensitivity) you will need to reduce the amount of gluten in your diet.

Gluten is the protein found in the grains wheat, rye, barley and triticale. Oats are frequently grown, harvested, milled and processed alongside gluten-containing grains, so they may be contaminated with gluten. They also contain a gluten-like protein which some people with coeliac disease react to. So, while research is ongoing, oats are currently not recommended for people with coeliac disease.

Understanding coeliac disease

We don't know how or why coeliac disease occurs, but it seems clear that both environment and genes play a part. For example, we do know that around 10 per cent of all parents, brothers, sisters or children (first-degree relatives) of someone with coeliac disease will also have it. And if one identical twin has coeliac disease, there is about a 70 per cent chance the other twin will also be affected.

We also know that it mainly affects Caucasians (people of European origin), but it is also known to occur in India and some Middle Eastern countries. It is rare in Asian and Australian Aboriginal populations.

We also now know it's not just an early childhood problem. Coeliac disease affects children and adults of any age. Many people only develop symptoms as adults and others have no obvious symptoms at all, making diagnosis very difficult. It is the most common and one of the most under-diagnosed hereditary autoimmune diseases.

In Australia and New Zealand, coeliac disease affects up to one in every hundred people. On top of this, for every person diagnosed with coeliac disease, there's likely to be another eight or nine undiagnosed people with symptoms or complications attributable to it.

If you have coeliac disease and you eat something that contains gluten, you will get an immune reaction in your small intestine. This damages your intestinal wall, reducing its ability to absorb nutrients from food and leading to deficiencies of the essential vitamins and minerals your body needs for growth, health, healing and energy. In children, if it's not diagnosed and treated, coeliac disease can affect growth and development. In adults, it can lead to long-term health problems including osteoporosis (due to calcium malabsorption), infertility, miscarriage, tooth decay and an increased risk of cancers of the digestive system.

Coeliac disease never goes away.

The good news is that you don't need drugs to deal with it, you can manage it effectively by following a strict gluten-free diet. By doing this, your intestinal wall will heal so nutrients can be absorbed, your symptoms will be resolved and long-term health problems may be prevented.

DIAGNOSING IT

Symptoms vary widely and some are very mild and non-specific. Some people have all or many of the symptoms while others may only have a few or none at all. Typical symptoms include:

- Fatigue, weakness and lethargy
- Low iron levels or unexplained anaemia that does not improve or recurs after taking iron supplements
- Wind, bloating and abdominal distension
- Stomach cramps
- Diarrhoea
- Constipation
- Nausea and vomiting
- Weight loss, and/or
- Poor weight gain, delayed growth and delayed puberty in children.

Some less common symptoms in adults include:

- Easy bruising of the skin
- Mouth ulcers
- Infertility and miscarriages
- Muscle spasms/cramps due to low calcium levels
- Deficiencies of vitamins B12, A, D, E and K

- Dental problems
- Poor memory and concentration, and
- Bone and joint pains.

If you have one or more of these signs or symptoms, make an appointment with your doctor for a check-up. They should refer you to a gastroenterologist who specialises in coeliac disease.

While blood tests that measure antibodies to gluten can be used to screen for coeliac disease, you actually need to have a small bowel biopsy to diagnose it. This test looks at whether the lining of the small intestine shows the typical damage known as villous atrophy (inflammation of the villi, which line the surface of the small intestine) seen in those with coeliac disease. A word of warning: it is important you don't jump the gun and start on a gluten-free diet before you have this test. If you do, the lining of your intestinal wall will repair and may not show up any damage when the biopsy is taken, thus preventing a proper diagnosis. Genetic testing can also be done to see if you have the genes which make you susceptible. A positive test doesn't necessarily mean you have coeliac disease but a negative test can rule it out and the test doesn't rely on eating gluten.

Understanding dermatitis herpetiformis

Dermatitis herpetiformis (DH) is also a genetic autoimmune disease caused by sensitivity to gluten. It causes an intensely itchy skin rash that looks like watery blisters or pimples. It generally presents in adult life and is more common in men than women and in people originally from some parts of northern Europe.

DH tends to appear over the kneecap, on the outer surface of the elbows, on the buttock area, around the ears, the shoulder blades, and in the hairline and eyebrows. It usually occurs symmetrically (on both sides of the body).

As with coeliac disease, you never get over it, but you can manage it successfully with a gluten-free diet.

DIAGNOSING IT

If you have DH, eating a food containing gluten triggers an immune response that deposits a chemical called immunoglobulin A (IgA) under the top layer of skin. Your dermatologist will need to take a skin biopsy to determine the presence of IgA deposits. Villous atrophy also occurs in people with DH.

It can take a year or two on a gluten free diet for the IgA deposits under the skin to clear completely. But don't despair, there are also good medications for providing immediate relief from the itching and burning rash.

Understanding gluten intolerance

Gluten intolerance is a broad term, which covers all kinds of sensitivity to gluten. In addition to those with coeliac disease and DH, there are many people who have a sensitivity to gluten who do not test positive for coeliac disease. These people have what is called non-coeliac gluten sensitivity, a condition in which the body does not tolerate large amounts of gluten.

If you have gluten intolerance you will generally need to reduce the amount of gluten in your diet but you probably won't have to follow a very strict gluten-free diet.

> A recent study from Monash University in Melbourne provided the first clear-cut evidence that gluten may induce irritable bowel syndrome like symptoms in people who *don't* have coeliac disease. Overall symptoms were significantly lower during the 6-week period in which the breads and muffins were gluten-free compared with the alternate period in which the breads and muffins were spiked with gluten.

DIAGNOSING IT

Symptoms of gluten intolerance may be similar to coeliac disease and commonly include digestive symptoms such as diarrhoea or constipation, wind and bloating.

The most accurate way to diagnose gluten intolerance is by doing an elimination diet – this involves removing foods containing gluten for a specified time to see if symptoms resolve, then reintroducing foods containing gluten to see if the symptoms recur. This should be done under the guidance of an Accredited Practising Dietitian (APD) who specialises in food allergies and intolerance. However, it is important to establish whether or not you have coeliac disease before you remove gluten from your diet.

Understanding wheat intolerance

In addition to gluten intolerance, some people have an intolerance to wheat but are able to tolerate other gluten-containing grains such as barley, rye and oats. Symptoms are similar to gluten intolerance and often include wind, bloating and constipation or diarrhoea.

DIAGNOSING IT

The most accurate way to diagnose wheat intolerance is by doing an elimination diet – this involves removing foods containing wheat for a specified period of time to see if the symptoms go away, then reintroducing foods containing wheat to see if the symptoms recur. Again, this should also be done under the guidance of an Accredited Practising Dietitian (APD) who specialises in food allergies and intolerances and, again, you should rule out coeliac disease before starting an elimination diet.

It is also possible to have an allergy to wheat although this is not common (it is more likely to be an intolerance) and is rarely as severe as other allergies such as those to nuts, egg and seafood. A wheat allergy can be diagnosed using skin prick testing – you should see your doctor if you suspect you might have an allergy to wheat.

Gluten-free diets and autism

Many parents with autistic children are trying them on a gluten-free, casein-free diet and we are hearing various reports of it helping. But so far it is not backed by research.

If you have a child with autism and decide to try a gluten-free diet we recommend working with an Accredited Practising Dietitian (APD) because eliminating gluten and casein means cutting out a large number of foods your child may have normally been eating. This can make it difficult to ensure that your child gets all the nutrients he or she needs, particularly while they are growing. Getting the right advice about what they can eat and making sure it is adequate to meet their nutritional needs for growth and development is essential.

Chapter 2: Gluten-free ground rules

Our ground rules cover what's in, what's out, what tends to be missing from a gluten-free diet and what you need to do about it.

While it may seem like mission impossible to suddenly change the way you shop, cook, feed the family and eat out, it's not the end of the world. There are plenty of great gluten-free foods to choose from. However, it may take more work and planning to start with.

In this chapter, we give you an idea of the sorts of foods you can enjoy to your heart's content, plus the ones you should leave off the menu. However, if you need to follow a strict gluten-free diet, we suggest as step one that you join your state coeliac society and take advantage of the up-to-date and comprehensive information they provide for their members on shopping, cooking and eating gluten-free. As for step two, it won't go amiss to brush up your food-label reading skills (see page 19).

> **Our favourite gluten-free food websites**
>
> www.coeliac.org.au
> www.glutenfreeshop.com.au
> www.coeliac.co.nz
> www.glutenfreegoodies.co.nz

What's in?

There are many more foods that you can eat than those that you can't. For starters, there are foods that are naturally gluten-free such as fruit and vegetables, legumes and nuts, many grains, meat, chicken and fish (providing they haven't been processed or crumbed). There's also an increasing number of packaged gluten-free foods such as breads, pastas and biscuits in supermarkets and health food stores that make following a gluten-free diet much easier. Some major supermarkets have a gluten-free section where you can shop with confidence, although if you have diabetes you will still need to check nutritional labels for things like fats and total carbs.

The following foods are suitable for those on a gluten-free diet:

- Rice, corn, buckwheat, millet, sorghum, quinoa, amaranth, polenta, tapioca, sago
- Gluten-free breads and breakfast cereals
- Gluten-free pasta, rice noodles and vermicelli, buckwheat noodles, bean thread noodles
- Pure corn taco shells and tortillas
- Legumes (dried peas, beans and lentils) – check canned varieties for gluten

- Plain nuts
- Fresh and frozen vegetables, salad vegetables
- Fresh, frozen, canned and dried fruit
- Fresh meat, chicken, fish, seafood, eggs and plain tofu
- Gluten-free sausages and processed meats
- Plain milk, cheese and yoghurt (flavoured varieties may contain gluten)
- Butter, margarine and oils (except for wheatgerm oil)
- Rice, corn, quinoa and buckwheat crackers and crispbreads
- Plain potato and corn chips; plain popcorn
- Gluten-free cakes and biscuits
- Plain chocolate
- Jam, marmalade, honey, tahini (sesame seed paste), peanut butter and other pure nut spreads
- Fresh and dried herbs and spices, salt and pepper (check dried herb and spice mixes for gluten)
- All types of vinegar apart from malt vinegar, and
- Water, soda water, mineral water, cordial, soft drinks, fruit and vegetable juices, plain cocoa, milk, tea, coffee, wine and spirits – but no beer (unless gluten-free), barley drinks or malted milk drinks.

What's out?

Wheat, rye, barley, oats and triticale, and foods made from these grains are out and need to be replaced with gluten-free alternatives. Gluten is also found in many foods that you might not think about (such as sauces, dressings, stock, spreads and processed meats), so it is important to become a label reader when shopping and to know exactly what to look for.

Here's a list (not definitive by any means) of foods that are out:

- Wheat (including semolina, couscous, spelt and burghul), rye, barley and triticale, and any foods made from these including breads, cereals, pasta, noodles, biscuits, cakes, muffins and flour
- Oats and foods containing oats, such as muesli and muesli bars
- Vegemite, Marmite and Promite
- Packaged stock (unless gluten-free)
- Many sauces, including soy sauce (unless gluten-free)
- Malt, barley malt, malt vinegar, breakfast cereals containing malt
- Textured Vegetable Protein (TVP) if derived from a gluten-containing grain
- Battered and crumbed foods, some commercial hot chips and potato wedges
- Beer, ale, stout (although gluten-free beer is now available)
- Maltodextrin from wheat (often found in soy milk, ice-cream and yoghurts, especially flavoured ones)
- Wheaten cornflour
- Baking powder (unless gluten-free)
- Some confectionery
- Licorice (although gluten-free licorice is now available)
- Many flavoured snacks including chips, corn chips and rice crackers
- Coffee substitutes (e.g. Ecco and Caro), malted milk drinks and flavours (e.g. Milo), beverage whitener, and
- Barley drinks.

What a gluten-free diet may miss and what you can do about it

Adults and children on a strict gluten-free diet can miss out on the numerous health benefits of:

- Getting enough fibre, and
- Managing blood glucose levels with low GI foods.

Cracking the gluten code on labels

Since the word gluten rarely appears on an ingredient list, you need to learn:

- Where less obvious sources of gluten may be found in foods
- Which ingredients are gluten-free, and
- Which are not.

You will need to make a habit of reading food labels every time you shop to ensure that what ends up in your trolley is safe for you to eat.

In Australia and New Zealand, the Foods Standards Code requires that:

- Food labelled as 'gluten-free' must not contain any detectable gluten and no oats or malt
- Food labelled as 'low gluten' must contain less than 0.02 per cent gluten (although these foods are not suitable for those on a gluten-free diet), and
- Ingredients derived from gluten-containing grains must always be declared on food labels.

ON A GLUTEN-FREE DIET YOU CAN MISS OUT ON FIBRE

You need about 30 grams of fibre a day for good bowel health. Filling, high fibre foods can also help you maintain a healthy weight by reducing hunger pangs. Plant foods are the only source of dietary fibre – it is found in the outer bran layers of grains, fruit, vegetables, nuts and legumes. There are two types of fibre – soluble and insoluble – and there is a difference.

Soluble fibres are the gel, gum and often jelly-like components of some foods, such as apples and legumes. By slowing down the time it takes for food to pass through the stomach and small intestine, soluble fibre can lower the glycemic response to a food. Good gluten-free sources include:

- Nuts and seeds
- Legumes (beans, peas and lentils)
- Apples and pears
- Strawberries and blueberries, and
- Psyllium.

Insoluble fibres are dry and bran-like and commonly called roughage. All cereal grains and products that retain the outer coat of the grain they are made from are sources of insoluble fibre, but not all foods containing insoluble fibre are low GI. Insoluble fibres will only lower the GI of a food when they exist in their original, intact form. An example is wholegrains, where the fibre acts as a physical barrier, delaying access of digestive enzymes and water to the starch within the cereal grain. Good gluten-free sources include:

- Whole kernel grains (such as brown rice, quinoa, buckwheat and millet)
- Nuts and seeds, and
- Most vegetables.

ON A GLUTEN-FREE DIET YOU CAN MISS OUT ON THE BENEFITS OF LOW GI FOODS

As we noted in the introduction, gluten-free diets tend to have a high GI. This is because low GI grain foods such as whole kernel breads, muesli, traditional porridge oats, pasta and barley are eliminated because they contain gluten, while the gluten-free alternative products are often quickly digested and absorbed, raising blood glucose and insulin levels.

Today we know that lowering the GI of your diet is one of the secrets to lifelong health. This is especially true for those people trying to prevent heart disease and type 2 diabetes. High GI foods tend to cause spikes in your blood glucose levels whereas foods with a low GI cause gentle rises. In Chapter 3 we look at carbohydrates, the GI and the lifelong benefits of low GI eating.

Chapter 3: Gluten free and low GI – why it matters

Today we know that it's important to be choosy about the type of carbohydrates we eat, because what we call their glycemic potency varies. This simply means that different carb foods will have dramatically different effects on blood glucose levels. The tool to use to help you choose the right type of carbs to trickle fuel into your engine and help you avoid the roller-coaster rise of 'sugar highs' followed by 'sugar lows' is the glycemic index, the GI.

The GI of a food reflects how fast its carbohydrates hit the bloodstream. It is based on scientific testing of real foods in real people, in the state in which they are normally consumed. It compares carbohydrates in different foods gram for gram. Foods with a low GI (55 and below) will have less of an effect on your blood glucose levels than eating foods with a high GI (70 and above).

- High GI carbohydrates break down rapidly during digestion, releasing glucose quickly into the bloodstream.

- Low GI carbohydrates break down slowly, releasing glucose gradually into the bloodstream.

The GI revolution

GI research has turned some widely held beliefs upside down. Historically, carbohydrates were described by their chemical structure: they were simple or complex. Sugars were simple and starches were complex for no better reason than sugars were small molecules and starches were big. By virtue of their size, complex carbohydrates were assumed to be the slowly digested goodies, causing only a small rise in blood glucose levels. Simple sugars, on the other hand, were assumed to be the villains of the piece – digested and absorbed quickly, producing a rapid rise in blood glucose.

But these were just assumptions. And research has proved them wrong. We now know that the concept of simple versus complex carbohydrates is not a useful or true guide to how carbohydrates behave inside our bodies. And that's why the GI caused a revolution.

Today we know the GI of hundreds of different food items that have been tested in healthy people (see the GI tables at the back of the book for some examples). The findings rocked the boat in many ways.

The first surprise was that the starch in foods such as white or highly processed bread, potatoes and many types of rice was digested and absorbed very quickly – not slowly, as had always been assumed.

Second, scientists found that the natural and refined sugars in foods such as fruit, dairy products and ice-cream did not produce more rapid or prolonged rises in blood glucose, as had always been thought. The truth was that most of the sugars in foods, regardless of the source, actually produced quite moderate blood glucose responses, lower than most of the starches. Why? Because sugars are a mixture of molecules, and some of them have only a very slight effect on blood glucose levels.

So this is why you need to forget the old distinctions between starchy foods and sugary foods, or simple versus complex carbohydrates. These concepts are no help at all when it comes to managing your blood glucose levels. By learning about the GI you can base your food choices on sound scientific evidence that will help you choose the right type of carbohydrates for your long-term health and wellbeing.

HOW CAN STARCHY FOODS BE DIGESTED QUICKLY?

As we said earlier, foods containing carbohydrates that break down quickly during digestion have the highest GI values. Most modern starchy foods, especially processed ones such as many types of breads and breakfast cereals (gluten-free or not), are high GI foods because the starch is fully gelatinised. This means it is highly soluble in digestive juices and easy for enzymes to attack. Because the digestion of starch produces its own weight as glucose, starchy foods can have a major impact on your blood glucose levels. Just like a flash flood when there's too much rain over a short space of time, rapid starch digestion results in blood glucose levels that rise quickly and create what you could call a 'metabolic flood'.

On the other hand, foods that contain carbohydrates that break down slowly, releasing glucose gradually into the bloodstream, have a low GI value. The starch in these foods is only partly gelatinised, and so it is more resistant to attack by digestive juices. The slow and steady digestion of low

GI foods produces a smoother blood glucose curve, greater feelings of fullness, and reduced metabolic disturbance. To show you the difference we have drawn a diagram – a picture can be worth a thousand words. The figure on page 28 shows the different effects of slow and fast carbohydrates on your blood glucose levels.

The most important factor that determines the GI of a food is the final physical state of the starch (not the sugars). If the starch granules have swollen and burst (think puffed and flaked cereal products), they will be digested in a flash, even if the fibre content is high. On the other hand, if the starch is still present in 'nature's packaging' (think whole intact grains and legumes), the process of digestion will take longer.

Over the last 50–100 years, advances in food processing – such as high-speed milling, high-pressure extrusion cooking and puffing technology – have had a profound effect on the carbohydrates we eat: they are much more rapidly digested and absorbed than the carbs our grandparents ate. It's one of the reasons why type 2 diabetes is far more common now than it was in the past.

But you don't have to eat only low GI carbs to get the health benefit. We know that when a low and a high GI food are combined in one meal (such as lentils and rice), the overall blood glucose response is between the two. You can keep both your glucose and your insulin levels lower over the course of a whole day if you choose at least one low GI food at each meal and for your snacks.

WHAT THIS MEANS FOR YOU AND YOUR HEALTH

Lowering your insulin levels is one of the secrets to lifelong health. High insulin levels caused by eating foods with a high GI are undesirable. In the long term they promote high blood fat, high blood glucose, high blood pressure and increase the risk of heart attack. Because of this, lowering the GI of your diet is significant in the long-term prevention of diabetes and heart disease and in improving your overall health. This is particularly relevant for anyone following a gluten-free diet – as we mentioned earlier in the book, gluten-free foods tend to have a higher GI. And if you have coeliac disease, a gluten-free diet is for life.

Eating a low GI diet has been scientifically proven to help people:

- With type 1 diabetes
- With type 2 diabetes
- With gestational diabetes (diabetes during pregnancy)
- Who are overweight
- Who are of normal weight but with excess abdominal fat
- Whose blood glucose levels are higher than desirable
- Who have been told they have pre-diabetes, 'impaired glucose tolerance' or a 'touch of diabetes'
- With high levels of triglycerides and low levels of HDL ('good') cholesterol
- With metabolic syndrome (the insulin resistance syndrome or syndrome X)
- Who suffer from polycystic ovarian syndrome (PCOS), and/or
- Who suffer from fatty liver disease (NAFLD or NASH).

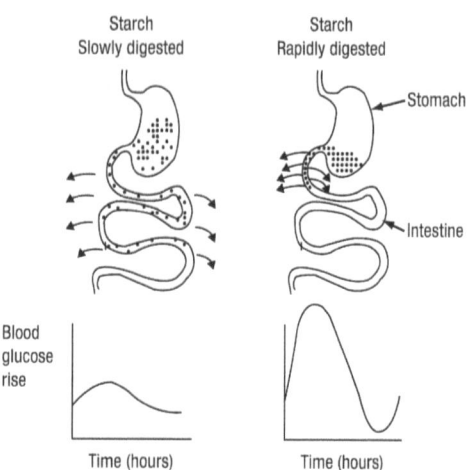

What happens when you eat foods containing carbohydrate

When you eat foods containing carbohydrate, such as bread, breakfast cereals, rice, pasta, noodles, starchy vegetables (such as potato) and fruit, your body converts them into a sugar called glucose during digestion. The glucose is absorbed from your intestine into your bloodstream and becomes the fuel that circulates around your body.

As the level of blood glucose rises after you have eaten a meal, your pancreas gets the message to release a powerful hormone called insulin. Insulin drives glucose out of your blood and into the cells. Once inside, glucose will be channelled into various pathways simultaneously – it will be used as an immediate source of energy, converted to glycogen (a storage form of glucose), or converted into fat. Insulin also turns off the use of fat as the cell's energy source.

Diabetes and the GI

About 10 per cent of people with coeliac disease also have type 1 diabetes and need to manage their blood glucose levels. But managing blood glucose levels is something we all need to do in our 'diabesity' world of expanding waistlines, because the higher the GI of your diet, the greater your risk of diabetes. Why? As we explained, foods with a high GI are digested quickly and cause a rapid rise in blood glucose and an outpouring of insulin. If you're constantly eating high GI meals you end up with chronically high insulin levels, which eventually lead to insulin resistance, where the cells that normally respond to insulin become insensitive to it, so your body thinks it has to make even more insulin.

All too often, type 2 diabetes is only diagnosed once the pancreas (which produces insulin) is absolutely worn out and cannot maintain sufficient insulin production to normalise blood glucose. Before you get to that point, eating a moderately high carbohydrate, low GI diet can actually improve the function of your pancreas and glycemic control, and can therefore prevent the onset of type 2 diabetes.

For people with type 2 diabetes, following a low GI diet can be as effective at lowering blood glucose as medication. A scientific analysis of 14 different studies from around the world of people with diabetes showed that low GI diets improved glycemic control significantly more than high GI or conventional diets. Improved glycemic control can prevent the onset and progression of diabetes complications.

On a daily basis, low GI foods can minimise the blood glucose peaks and troughs that make life so difficult for people with diabetes. Since they are slowly digested and absorbed, low GI foods reduce insulin demand – lessening the strain on the struggling pancreas of a person with type 2 diabetes and potentially lowering insulin requirements for those with type 1 diabetes. Lower insulin levels have the follow-on benefit of reducing the risk of large blood vessel damage, thus reducing the risk of developing heart disease.

Heart health and the GI

These days, most of us are well aware of the importance of cutting back on saturated fat and choosing 'good fats' for heart health. We now know that the higher the GI of your diet the greater your risk of heart disease. This is because a high level of glucose in the blood means:

- More glucose moves into cells lining the arteries, which causes inflammation, thickening and stiffening of artery walls, so the blood vessels lose their elasticity
- Highly reactive, charged particles called 'free radicals' (like 'sparks') are formed and these destroy the machinery inside the cell, eventually causing the cell to wither and die
- Glucose sticks to cholesterol in the blood which promotes the formation of fatty plaque and prevents the body from breaking down excess cholesterol, and
- Higher levels of insulin are present, which raises blood pressure and blood fats, while suppressing 'good' (HDL) cholesterol levels.

On the other hand, a diet rich in slowly digested, low GI carbs, along with regular exercise, will reduce your risk of heart disease. By lowering your blood glucose after meals and reducing high insulin levels, you'll have:

- Healthier blood vessels that are more elastic, dilate more easily and aid blood flow
- Thinner blood and improved blood flow
- More potential for weight loss and therefore less pressure on the heart, and
- Better blood fats – more of the good cholesterol and less of the bad.

Weight loss, the GI and satisfying hunger

There is no doubt that reducing portion sizes and eating fewer kilojoules will lead to weight loss. These days, we are eating less fat but getting fatter. Instead of eating fewer kilojoules we are eating more, especially in the form of high GI, refined starches and sugars. The real solution to both weight loss and weight maintenance is to be choosy about the type of carbs you eat. Here are some reasons why:

- Eating high GI carbs causes a surge of glucose in the blood. Although the body needs glucose it doesn't need this much all in one hit, so it secretes insulin to move the glucose out of the blood and store it in the cells. This drives blood glucose levels down and directs all incoming food to storage – glucose to glycogen and fat, and fats to fat storage
- The action of insulin means blood glucose levels begin to decline rapidly

- The brain detects falling blood glucose and, because it relies solely on glucose to keep us alive, it sends out hunger signals
- The body would normally respond by releasing stored glucose for energy, but if insulin levels remain elevated (as they do in insulin resistance), the release of stored fuel is inhibited, and
- Low levels of fuel and high levels of insulin can then trigger the release of stress hormones such as adrenaline which scour the blood for more glucose. This can translate to hunger, light-headedness and feeling shaky. The only way to relieve the state of hunger is with another snack.

If you feel hungry all the time, here's how and why low GI foods can help you turn off the switch:

- Low GI foods are rich in carbohydrate – a far superior appetite suppressant than fat
- Many low GI foods are less processed, which means they require more chewing, helping to signal satiety (fullness) to your brain
- Low GI foods are often accompanied by fibre, so they create a greater feeling of fullness in your stomach
- They are more slowly digested, which means they stay in your intestines for longer, keeping you feeling satisfied
- They trickle glucose into your bloodstream slowly, helping you avoid the roller-coaster ride in blood glucose levels (a cycle of 'sugar highs' followed by 'sugar lows'), and

- Low GI foods help overcome the body's natural tendency to slow down kilojoule burning (metabolic rate) while dieting.

Managing PCOS and the GI

Polycystic ovarian syndrome (PCOS) is thought to affect 5–10 per cent of women in developed countries. Characteristics of the syndrome can include irregular periods, infertility, heavy body-hair growth, acne, excess weight gain and difficulties losing weight. In many women it goes undiagnosed because the symptoms may be subtle, such as faint facial hair. Women with PCOS are also at higher risk of developing diabetes and cardiovascular disease.

Insulin resistance – where the body resists the normal actions of the hormone insulin – is at the root of PCOS and that's where the GI comes in. To overcome insulin resistance the body secretes more insulin than normal. Among other effects, high insulin levels cause an increased production of testosterone (male hormones) by the ovaries, causing a host of hormonal imbalances.

To manage PCOS symptoms effectively you need to make the change to low GI eating and build more activity into your life. The benefits will include:

- Reducing PCOS symptoms
- Achieving and maintaining healthy weight
- Controlling blood glucose and insulin levels
- Boosting fertility, and
- Gaining control and quality of life.

The GI and pregnancy

Pregnancy is a stage in life when the carbohydrates in food play a starring role. This is because the mother's average blood glucose level throughout the day is directly correlated with your baby's growth rate *in the womb*. Quite simply, glucose is the primary fuel that drives all aspects of the baby's development. If glucose levels are too high, then the baby will grow too fast and be born with excessive amounts of body fat. This is not a new finding. It's the main reason why women who have type 1 diabetes (a condition that requires daily insulin injections to maintain normal glucose levels) are given close medical attention before and during their pregnancies. It's also the principal reason why all pregnant women are routinely screened at 26–28 weeks' gestation to determine if they have developed gestational diabetes. What's new is that we now know that even mildly elevated glucose levels during pregnancy have serious consequences.

Infant birth weights and child obesity have increased hand in hand over recent decades in most industrialised nations. We now know that life inside the womb is a critical period for the metabolic 'programming' of obesity in later life. A mother's weight at the time of conception, and weight gain from early to late pregnancy, profoundly influence her infant's birth weight and future risk of becoming overweight. Reducing the GI of the diet is one of the safest and most effective ways of ensuring that the baby grows at the optimum rate, without laying down excessive body fat. In our newest book, *The Bump to Baby Diet: Low GI Eating Plan for a Healthy Pregnancy*, we tell the full story.

Why insulin resistance is a problem

Elevations in blood glucose after eating high GI foods are followed by elevations in insulin. When insulin levels are frequently raised the cells that usually respond to insulin become resistant to its signals. This means that glucose hangs around in the bloodstream at higher than normal concentrations, where it can damage cells.

A low GI diet is invaluable in the management of insulin resistance because it will:
- Result in lower blood glucose after meals, and thereby
- Reduce the demand for insulin, which can
- Help appetite control and improve weight loss.

Chapter 4: Your low GI, gluten-free food finder

Low GI foods form the basis of a healthy diet. It is the way nature intended us to eat – low fat, nutritious foods that satisfy hunger. Even on a wheat-free or gluten-free diet, you'll find that there are many low GI gluten-free foods you can enjoy in four of the five food groups:

- Virtually all fruits and vegetables
- Whole kernel grains in the breads and cereals group
- Legumes of all types in the meat and alternatives group, and
- Milk and yoghurt among the dairy foods.

Which fruits and vegetables to choose

Temperate climate fruits – apples, pears, citrus (oranges, grapefruit) and stone fruits (peaches, plums, apricots) – all have low GI values.

Tropical fruits such as pineapple, pawpaw, rockmelon and watermelon tend to have higher GI values, but their glycemic load (we explain this on page 44) is low because they are low in carbohydrate. Bananas (so long as they are not overripe) have a low GI. So you can enjoy these tropical fruits in season, as they are excellent sources of antioxidants.

Think of vegetables as 'free' foods – they are full of fibre, essential nutrients and protective antioxidants that will fill you up without adding extra kilojoules. Most are so low in carbohydrate they have no measurable effect on your blood glucose levels at all. In fact, leafy green and salad vegetables have so little carbohydrate that we can't test their GI. Even in generous serving sizes they will have no effect on your blood glucose levels.

Higher carbohydrate starchy vegetables include sweetcorn (which is actually a cereal grain), potato, sweet potato, taro and yam, so watch the portion sizes with these.

Most varieties of potatoes sold in Australia have a high GI. The exceptions are Carisma (GI 55), Nicola (GI 58) and baby new (chat) potatoes (GI 65). Carisma potatoes are a newly released variety with a firm texture that is ideal for potato salads but still appropriate for other uses. To ensure a low GI result, use the 'quick' cooking method of placing 1 cm-thick slices of unpeeled potatoes in hot (not boiling) water, then bringing to the boil and cooking for approximately 4 minutes until 'al dente'. Potatoes should be firm but not cooked through. Carisma potatoes are sold exclusively through Coles supermarkets. (See www.carismapotatoes.com.au for more information.)

Pumpkin, carrots, peas, parsnips and beetroot contain some carbohydrate, but a normal serving size contains so little that it won't raise your blood glucose levels significantly.

Which breads and cereals to choose

The key is to look for less processed or refined products if you can – the ones with lots of wholegrain kernels and fibre. Remember, the whole point is to get your stomach to do the processing. Slowly.

There are a number of gluten-free breads, breakfast cereals, snack foods and pastas on the market. As not many have been GI tested, here are some guidelines for selecting lower GI options.

BREAD

At the time of publication, we found only one low GI gluten-free bread on the supermarket shelves – Country Life Low GI Gluten Free bread (GI 53).

Most of the gluten-free breads, including rolls and wraps, tested have been found to have a high GI. But here is a tip: check out the ingredients list and opt for breads that include chickpea- or legume-based flours and psyllium. For example, we know that chapattis made with besan (chickpea flour) have a low GI. If you make your own bread, try adding buckwheat kernels, rice bran and psyllium husks to lower the GI.

If you like tortillas as a wrap, Diego's White Corn Tortillas (GI 53) and Woolworth's Select White Corn Tortillas (GI 53) are both gluten-free and low GI.

BREAKFAST CEREALS

Freedom Foods Muesli has a low GI. Rice bran and buckwheat kernels also have a low GI and can be used with other ingredients to make your own gluten-free muesli. See our recipe on page 97.

Most gluten-free breakfast cereals, including rice, buckwheat or millet puffs and flakes, have a moderate or high GI because they are refined, not wholegrain, foods. But you can reduce the GI if you serve them with fruit and yoghurt and a teaspoon or two of psyllium to boost the fibre.

If you like cooked cereal, try quinoa porridge (made from whole quinoa grains) or make your own rice porridge (from a lower GI rice). Add psyllium husks and rice bran, along with fruit and low fat milk or yoghurt. Again, see our recipes on pages 103–4.

NOODLES AND PASTA

There are several low GI, gluten-free options available in both fresh and dried varieties:

- Buckwheat (soba) noodles
- Cellophane noodles, also known as Lungkow bean thread noodles or green bean vermicelli, made from mung bean flour, and
- Rice noodles, made from ground or pounded rice flour.

Most gluten-free pastas based on rice and corn (maize) tend to have moderate to high GI values. So opt for pastas made from legumes or soy – although they may be harder to find.

Pasta is best eaten al dente (firm to the bite). It should be slightly firm and offer some resistance when you are chewing it. Al dente pasta has a lower GI, too, as overcooking boosts the GI. Although most manufacturers specify a cooking time on the packet, don't take their word for it. Start testing about 2–3 minutes before the indicated cooking time is up.

You can further reduce the overall GI of your pasta meal by serving it (hot or cold) with sauces and salsas that contain some vegetables or legumes. See how we do it in our recipes in the Salads and Soups section (pages 141–158) and in the Mains section (pages 159–180).

WHOLE CEREAL GRAINS

Low GI cereal grains for those on a gluten-free diet include buckwheat, quinoa, some varieties of rice (see below) and sweetcorn. Currently there are no published values for amaranth, sorghum and teff. Millet has a high GI.

RICE

Rice can have a very high GI value, or a moderate one, depending on the variety and its amylose content. Amylose is a kind of starch that resists gelatinisation. Although rice is a wholegrain food, when it's cooked, the millions of microscopic cracks in the grains let water penetrate right to the middle of the grain, allowing the starch granules to swell and become fully 'gelatinised', thus very easy to digest. Instant and quick cooking rices all tend to have a high GI.

So, if you are a big rice eater, opt for the lower GI varieties with a higher amylose content such as basmati rice (GI 58), SunRice Doongara CleverRice™ (GI 54), or Moolgiri medium grain rice (GI 54). You'll also find a number of lower GI rice varieties on the database at www.glycemicindex.com or in the latest *Low GI Diet Shopper's Guide to GI Values* – there's an updated edition each year.

Brown rice is an extremely nutritious form of rice and contains several B-group vitamins, minerals, dietary fibre and protein. The varieties tested to date tend to have a moderate or high GI, so try to combine this nourishing food with low GI ingredients like lentils or beans, or even in combination with wild rice. Wild rice (GI 57) is not rice at all, but a type of grass seed. Arborio rice, used mainly in risotto, releases its starch during cooking and has a medium GI.

> ### What about oats?
>
> To recommend that people with coeliac disease avoid oats is controversial because some have been able to eat certain amounts of oats without any damage to their intestinal wall. Oats can add soluble fibre and nutrients to a gluten-free diet. Scientists are currently studying whether people with coeliac disease can tolerate oats. Until the studies are complete, people with coeliac disease should follow their physician's or dietitian's advice about eating oats.

LEGUMES (PULSES)

Dried or canned legumes including beans, chickpeas and lentils are among nature's lowest GI foods. They are high in fibre and packed with nutrients, providing protein, carbohydrate, B vitamins, folate and minerals. Check canned varieties for gluten content.

When you add legumes to meals and snacks, you reduce the overall GI of your diet because your body digests them slowly. This is primarily because their starch breaks down relatively slowly (or incompletely) during cooking and they contain tannins and enzyme inhibitors that also slow digestion. So make the most of beans, chickpeas, lentils, and whole and split dried peas. You'll find we use them in many of our recipes – even cakes.

NUTS

Although nuts are high in fat (averaging around 50 per cent of their content), it is largely unsaturated, so they make a healthy substitute for snacks such as biscuits, cakes, pastries, potato chips and chocolate. They also contain relatively little carbohydrate, so most do not have a GI value. Those which have been tested (including peanuts, pecans, cashews and mixed nuts) have very low GI values. Avoid the varieties that are salted and cooked in oil – choose raw and unsalted. Also be aware that dry-roasted nuts may contain gluten.

Chestnuts are quite different from other nuts in that they are low in fat and higher in carbohydrate. Naturally gluten-free, they have recently been found to have a low GI, which makes them a great low GI, high fibre carbohydrate food for people with coeliac disease. Roasted chestnuts are a nutritious snack or addition to meals and can also be ground into a flour for making breads, cakes and pasta.

LOW FAT DAIRY FOODS AND CALCIUM-ENRICHED SOY PRODUCTS

Low fat varieties of milk, yoghurt and ice-cream, or calcium-enriched soy alternatives, provide you with sustained energy, boosting your calcium intake but not your saturated fat intake. Check the labels of yoghurts, ice-creams and soy milks as some contain wheat-based maltodextrins or barley malt, which should be avoided.

Cheese is a good source of calcium, but it is a protein food not a carbohydrate as its lactose is drawn off in the whey during production. This means that GI is not relevant to cheese. Although perfect for sandwich fillings, snacks and toppings for gratin dishes, remember that cheese can also contribute a fair number of kilojoules. Most cheese is around 30 per cent fat, much of it saturated. Ricotta and cottage cheese are good low fat choices.

What's glycemic load?

Your blood glucose rises and falls when you eat a meal containing carbs. How high it rises and how long it remains high depends on the quality of the carbs (the GI) and the quantity. Glycemic load, or GL, combines both the quality and quantity of carbohydrate in one 'number'. The formula for calculating the GL of a particular meal is:

GL = (GI × the amount of carbohydrate) divided by 100

Although the GL concept has been useful in scientific research, it's the GI that has proven most helpful to people with diabetes. That's because a diet with a low GL, unfortunately, can be mixed – full of healthy low GI carbs in some cases, but too low in carbs and full of the wrong sorts of fats, such as fatty meat and butter, in others.

If you choose healthy low GI foods – at least one in each meal and monitor the amount of carbohydrate – chances are you'll be on the right track to blood glucose control.

Part 2

How do you do it?

The best type of eating plan for most of us, including anyone on a gluten-free diet, is one that is low in saturated fat and contains sufficient protein and moderate amounts of carbohydrate, with most of the carbohydrate choices being low GI. It should have plenty of vegetables, salads, fruit, legumes and wholegrains. Here, we give you some tips on how to make the switch to low GI, gluten-free eating along with 7-day menus for adults, children and vegetarians to help you and your family get started.

Chapter 5: Going gluten-free and low GI

Healthy gluten-free eating guidelines

Every day:

1. Eat seven or more servings of fruit and vegetables (at least five servings of vegetables and two of fruit)
2. Opt for gluten-free whole kernel grain breads and cereals with a low GI
3. Eat more legumes (dried beans, peas and lentils)
4. Include nuts and seeds regularly in your diet
5. Choose lean meats, omega-3-enriched eggs and low fat dairy products or calcium-enriched alternatives
6. Eat more fish and seafood, and
7. Opt for monounsaturated and omega-3 polyunsaturated fats such as olive and canola oil, and those found in fish, nuts, seeds and avocado.

1. Eat seven or more servings of fruit and vegetables

Fruit and vegetables should form a major part of any healthy eating plan. They are rich sources of vitamins, minerals, antioxidants and phytochemicals, all of which are important for good health and can help to protect you against diseases such as cancer and cardiovascular disease. They are high in fibre and (apart from avocados and olives, which contain 'healthy' monounsaturated fats) are very low in fat.

Variety is the key. Don't just stick with your favourites (apples, bananas, oranges) or the same old vegetable varieties, such as beans, carrots and peas. Why not buy something different each time you shop? Aim to make your plate or fruit bowl as colourful as possible. Ask your greengrocer what's in season right now.

Fruit – what's a serve?

One serve is equivalent to:
- 1 medium piece (about 120 g) of fresh fruit, such as an apple, banana, mango, orange, peach or pear
- 2 small pieces (about 60 g each) of fresh fruit, such as apricots, kiwi fruit or plums
- 1 cup of fresh diced or canned fruit pieces including grapes, berries and strawberries
- 4–5 (about 30 g) dried apricot halves, apple rings, figs or prunes
- 1½ tablespoons (about 30 g) sultanas
- 200 ml of 100 per cent fruit juice, homemade or unsweetened

How much a day?
- Smaller eaters: 2 serves
- Medium eaters: 3 serves
- Bigger eaters: 4 serves

Vegetables – what's a serve?
One serve is equivalent to:
- ½ cup (about 80 g) cooked vegetables (other than starchy vegetables – potato, sweetcorn and sweet potato)
- 1 cup raw salad vegetables
- 1 cup (250 ml) vegetable soup (without cream!)
- 1 cup (250 ml) pure vegetable juice

How much a day?
Even the smallest eater should aim to eat five or more serves of vegetables every day, including fresh and frozen vegetables, vegetable juices and soups. This is a minimum of 2½ cups of cooked vegetables or 4 cups of salad.

Starchy vegetables – what's a serve?
Starchy vegetables such as sweet potato, potato and sweetcorn are higher in carbohydrate, so their GI and serve size is more relevant. One serve is equivalent to:
- 1 medium (120 g) potato (slightly smaller than a tennis ball)
- ½ cup mashed potato
- 120 g sweet potato
- ½ cup sweetcorn kernels
- ½ cob sweetcorn
- 80 g taro or yam
- 1 large (160 g) parsnip

How much a day?

The following is recommended in addition to the five or more vegetable servings:

- Smaller eaters: 1 serve
- Medium eaters: 3 serves
- Bigger eaters: 4 serves

GET YOUR SEVEN SERVES A DAY

Breakfast

- Include fruit (fresh, canned in natural juice, or dried) with your breakfast cereal.
- Try a fresh fruit smoothie for a quick but satisfying breakfast meal.
- For a more substantial breakfast, add some vegetables on your low GI, gluten-free toast – try asparagus, mushrooms, tomato and onion, or sliced tomato and avocado.
- Mushrooms, asparagus and tomato are also great added to omelettes.

Lunch

- On your gluten-free sandwich, add plenty of salad vegetables, such as tomato, lettuce, cucumber, sprouts, beetroot, grated carrot and capsicum.
- Try the same with toasted sandwiches. Go for tomato, capsicum, mushroom, sweet potato, olives, zucchini and eggplant.
- Use avocado as a spread on your sandwich instead of butter.
- Salads are a great way to fill up at lunchtime and the combinations are endless. Don't stick with lettuce, tomato and cucumber, try adding snow peas, capsicum,

sweetcorn, green beans, steamed broccoli, asparagus, roasted sweet potato and eggplant, sundried tomatoes and a few cubes of avocado or some olives.
- During colder weather, soups are a great way to get more vegetables into your diet. Try pumpkin, sweet potato, lentil, split pea, minestrone or tomato.

Dinner
- Include vegetables or salads with all main meals. Serve them steamed, seasoned with fresh or dried herbs, or with a dressing made from olive oil, lemon juice, balsamic vinegar and garlic.
- Always have some frozen vegetables handy for when you don't have time to shop for fresh varieties.
- If you don't like vegetables on their own, add them to stir-fries, curries, casseroles and grated into mince.
- Choose vegetable-based dishes when eating out or ask for a side salad with your meal.

Snacks and desserts
- Fruit and grated vegetables such as carrot and zucchini can be added into cakes and muffins.
- Choose fruit for snacks. It's widely available, inexpensive, easy to eat, and without the added fat and sugar found in many other snack foods.
- Serve raw vegetables such as celery, carrot, cucumber, capsicum, broccoli or cauliflower florets as a snack served with a low fat dip or salsa.
- Make fruit the basis of your desserts. Try baked apples, fruit crumbles and tinned fruit with low fat custard, yoghurt or ice-cream.

2. Opt for gluten-free whole kernel grain breads and cereals with a low GI

Whole kernel grain breads and cereals have many health benefits. Most have a lower GI than refined cereal grains and they are also nutritionally superior, containing higher levels of fibre, vitamins, minerals and phytochemicals. We know from studies that a higher consumption of cereal fibre and wholegrains is associated with a reduced incidence of type 2 diabetes, cancer and heart disease.

Eating these higher fibre foods can help you lose weight, too, because they fill you up sooner and leave you feeling full for longer. They also improve insulin sensitivity and lower insulin levels. When this happens, your body makes more use of fat as a source of fuel. What could be better when you are trying to lose weight?

Replacing processed grains and cereals for those with a lower GI is a key part of making the change to a healthy, low GI diet.

Breads and cereals – what's a serve?

One serve is equivalent to:
- 1 slice gluten-free bread (sandwich thickness) or ½ gluten-free bread roll
- ½ cup (30 g) gluten-free breakfast cereal or muesli
- ½ cup cooked rice or other small gluten-free grains such as quinoa; or cooked gluten-free pasta or noodles

How much a day?
- Smaller eaters: 4 serves
- Medium eaters: 6 serves
- Bigger eaters: 8 serves

> **Watch that glucose load with rice, noodles and pasta**
>
> It's all too easy to overeat these foods, so keep portions moderate. Even if it has a low GI value, eating too much will have a marked effect on your blood glucose. So, instead of piling your plate with rice, noodles or pasta, fill it with vegetables and a little meat, chicken, fish or tofu. For example, a cup of rice combined with plenty of mixed vegetables and a little protein food can turn into three cups of a rice-based meal and fit easily into any adult's daily diet.

ENJOY MORE GLUTEN-FREE BREADS AND CEREALS
Breakfast
- For sweetness, add some stewed apple, a few sultanas and a sprinkle of cinnamon to quinoa or brown rice porridge. Top with low fat milk or soy milk.
- In warmer weather, choose gluten-free cereals based on rice bran, psyllium and buckwheat, or use these grains to make your own muesli (see recipe page 97).
- For those who prefer toast, choose gluten-free wholegrain varieties and those labelled low GI or carrying the GI symbol.

Lunch
- For sandwiches, go for wholegrain gluten-free breads and wraps.
- Buckwheat or quinoa can be used to make gluten-free tabbouli to add to wraps and sandwiches.
- Rice vermicelli noodles can be added to Thai salads, rice paper rolls or Asian soups.

Dinner

- Choose Asian noodles such as rice, bean thread or soba (buckwheat) noodles in place of rice, but always check that they are completely gluten-free.
- Try lower GI rices such as basmati, SunRice Doongara CleverRice™ and Moolgiri medium grain rice.
- Buckwheat and quinoa can be added to soups and casseroles or used to make salads.

Snacks and desserts

- Gluten-free fruit loaf with ricotta makes a satisfying snack for those with a sweet tooth.
- Make muffins using rice bran, buckwheat and psyllium husks, fruit or dried fruit, and nuts or almond meal.
- For dessert, you could try a fruit crumble topped with rice bran cereal or a suitable crushed low GI gluten-free cereal, or creamed rice made with a low or lower GI rice.

3. Eat more legumes

Legumes are high in fibre – both soluble and insoluble. They are also packed with nutrients, providing a valuable source of protein, carbohydrate, B vitamins, folate and minerals. Sprouted dried beans such as mung, soy, chickpeas and lentils, are excellent sources of vitamin C, and are great eaten raw in a salad or stir-fried.

Legumes are an important part of the healthy, low GI way of eating. They're particularly important for those on a gluten-free diet as they can provide much of the fibre and nutrients found in the gluten-containing grains that you can no longer eat. Try to put them on the menu at least twice a week – more often if you are vegetarian.

What are legumes?

Legumes (also known as pulses) are the edible dried seeds – such as beans, peas and lentils – found inside the mature pods of leguminous plants. Nutritionally, they are quite different from fresh, young green beans and peas, which don't have as much protein or fibre because of their high water content.

Thanks to their tendency to cause intestinal gas, there has been a bad odour about legumes, and lots of jokes. But not all legumes make you windy and not everyone has the problem. Cooking legumes in fresh water (not in the water you soaked them in) and rinsing the canned varieties helps. Eat them regularly – it can improve your tolerance.

Canned legumes are ready to use, and only need heating through. Meals based on these are much faster to prepare than meat-based meals, but check the label for wheat-based thickeners – these should be avoided.

Tofu (soy bean curd) is an easy way of using soy beans. It has a mild flavour, but absorbs the flavours of other foods, making it delicious when it has been marinated in tamari, ginger and garlic and tossed into a stir-fry. Tofu contains very little carbohydrate, so it doesn't have a GI.

Legumes – what's a serve?
- One serve is equivalent to ½ cup of cooked beans, lentils, chickpeas or cooked whole dried or split peas.

How much a week?
- Incorporate legumes into your meals at least twice a week as a starchy vegetable – more often if you are a vegetarian.

HOW YOU CAN MAKE THESE 'SUPERFOODS' A REGULAR PART OF YOUR LOW GI DIET

Breakfast
- Baked beans on gluten-free toast make an easy and satisfying breakfast.
- Try scrambling silken tofu in place of eggs. Add some fresh or dried herbs and chopped tomato, and sauté in a little olive oil.

Lunch
- Lentil, split pea or minestrone soup all make a satisfying winter lunch.
- Baked bean toasted sandwiches on gluten-free bread are an easy all-time favourite.
- Add a can of three-bean mix or some chickpeas to a salad to really fill you up.
- Lentils or chickpeas can be made into burgers, served on a gluten-free roll or wrap.
- Spread hommous (made from chickpeas) on your gluten-free sandwich or wrap in place of butter.

Dinner

- Add red kidney beans to mince and serve with tacos, burritos, gluten-free pasta or rice.
- Chickpeas have a nutty flavour and team well with curries and stir-fries.
- Make some dahl (lentils or split peas cooked with spices) as an accompaniment to your next curry.
- Green soy beans (edamame) are a tasty addition to a stir-fry. They are available frozen from most Asian grocery stores.
- Add cannellini, borlotti or black eye beans to stews and casseroles.
- Firm tofu can be cubed, marinated and added to stir-fries or threaded onto skewers with vegetables to make kebabs for the barbecue or grill.
- Substitute canned lentils for some of the mince in spaghetti bolognaise or a meat loaf.

Snacks and desserts

- Silken tofu can be used in place of cream cheese to make desserts such as cheesecake.
- Roasted chickpeas or soy beans (dubbed chicknuts and soynuts) make a tasty and satisfying snack.
- If you are really hungry, try a small tin of baked beans or four-bean mix as a snack.
- For a healthy dip, go for hommous or bean purée with carrot and celery sticks.

> ## Cooking with legumes
>
> **Dried legumes** Dried beans and peas need soaking and cooking before you use them in your meals. Lentils and split peas cook much faster and don't need soaking.
>
> - To soak beans, rinse and place them in a saucepan and cover with two to three times their volume of cold water. Set aside to soak overnight or throughout the day. If time is limited, take a shortcut by adding three times the volume of water to rinsed beans, bring to a boil for a few minutes, then remove from heat, and set aside to soak for an hour.
> - To cook, drain off the soaking water, add fresh water, and bring to the boil, then simmer until beans are tender. Use the directions on the packet as a time guide.
> - Don't add salt to the cooking water. It slows down water absorption, increasing cooking time.
> - Don't cook beans in the water they have soaked in. Substances that contribute to flatulence are leached from the beans into the soaking and cooking waters.
>
> **Canned legumes** Most legumes are available canned, making cooking with beans quick and easy. One 400 g can of beans substitutes for ¾ cup of dried beans. Check the label to avoid those with wheat-based thickeners.

4. Include nuts and seeds regularly in your diet

Like legumes, nuts are a good food to include regularly. They are high in fibre and contain a range of important vitamins and minerals that can be harder to get on a gluten-free diet. They are a healthy choice because they contain:

- Very little saturated fat (the fats are predominantly mono- or polyunsaturated)
- Dietary fibre
- Vitamin E, an antioxidant believed to help prevent heart disease, and
- Folate, copper and magnesium, nutrients thought to protect against heart disease.

Walnuts and pecans also contain some omega-3 fats, while linseeds are very rich in omega-3s, lignans and plant oestrogens. When freshly ground, linseeds have a subtle nutty flavour, making them a great addition to breads, muffins, biscuits and cereals.

Remember to choose the unsalted variety – salted nuts are usually roasted in saturated fat. And stick to a handful a day if you are watching your weight.

Nuts – what's a serve?

One serve provides 10 g of fat (apart from chestnuts which are almost fat-free) and is equivalent to:
- 15 g (about 10 small or 5 large) nuts
- 1 tablespoon of seeds
- 3 teaspoons (15 ml) peanut butter or nut spread

How much a day?

Aim for a small handful (no fingers) of nuts most days.
- Smaller eaters: 1 serve most days
- Medium eaters: 1 serve a day
- Bigger eaters: 1–2 serves most days

EASY WAYS TO EAT MORE NUTS AND SEEDS
Breakfast
- Sprinkle a mixture of nuts and seeds over your cereal.
- Use a spread such as peanut, almond or cashew butter on your toast in place of butter or margarine.

Lunch
- Add a handful of walnuts or pine nuts to your salad.
- Tahini (sesame seed paste) can be used as a spread on sandwiches or in salads in place of mayonnaise.

Dinner
- Add nuts and seeds to your favourite meals – try peanuts or sesame seeds in a stir-fry, cashews in a curry, crushed macadamias with fish or chicken, or roasted chestnuts with pasta.
- Pesto (ground pine nuts with basil, garlic and olive oil) makes a good pasta sauce or accompaniment to meat or fish.
- Tahini can be used as an alternative to sour cream on potatoes or drizzled over roasted vegetables.

Snacks and desserts
- Enjoy nuts as a snack. Just be careful not to eat too many. Limit them to one small handful (about 15 g) each day.
- Gluten-free crackers, rice cakes or toast with nut spread make a satisfying snack.
- Nuts and seeds can be added to baked goods. Try walnuts, hazelnuts, almond meal and ground chestnuts in cakes and muffins, and sunflower seeds, pepitas (pumpkin seeds), sesame seeds and linseeds in bread.

5. Choose lean meats, omega-3 eggs and low fat dairy

Reducing your intake of saturated fat doesn't mean that you need to avoid red meat and dairy products. They are good sources of protein, iron and calcium.

If you enjoy meat, we suggest eating lean red meat two or three times a week, and accompanying it with salad and vegetables. Trim all visible fat from meat and remove the skin (and the fat just below it) from chicken. Game meat such as rabbit and venison are not only lean but are also good sources of omega-3 fatty acids. So are organ meats such as liver and kidney. If you choose not to eat red meat or are trying to reduce your intake, legumes and tofu are good alternatives. They can provide the protein, iron and zinc also found in red meat.

Replacing full-fat dairy foods with reduced-fat, low fat or fat-free varieties will also help you reduce your overall saturated fat intake. Dairy products, including milk, yoghurt and cheese, are among the richest sources of calcium in our diet, provide protein, and a number of important vitamins and minerals such as vitamin B12, phosphorus, magnesium and zinc.

If you are lactose intolerant, or prefer not to eat dairy products, you could choose calcium-fortified soy products such as soy milk and soy yoghurt. Soy products contain mostly polyunsaturated fat and the protein in soy products can help to lower cholesterol levels. They are also a source of omega-3 fatty acids and phytoestrogens. However, check the labels on these products as some soy milks contain gluten, usually derived from wheat-based maltodextrin.

What about eggs and cholesterol? We used to think that eating high-cholesterol foods such as eggs, prawns and other shellfish would raise our blood cholesterol levels. We now know that our liver compensates for the increased cholesterol intake by reducing cholesterol production. This means that most people could eat an egg a day, for example, without harming their heart. However, a small percentage of people have an inherited condition called familial hypercholesterolemia, which impairs this self-regulation.

To enhance your intake of omega-3 fats, we suggest that you eat omega-3-enriched eggs if you can find them. These enriched eggs are produced by feeding hens a diet (including canola and linseeds) that is naturally rich in omega-3s.

Lean meat, chicken and eggs – what's a serve?

One serve is equivalent to:
- 100 g raw lean meat or chicken
- 2 medium eggs
- 1 small chop, visible fat trimmed
- ½ cup cooked lean mince
- ½ skinless chicken breast
- 1 large chicken drumstick

How much a day?

Although they're nutritious, meat, chicken and eggs do not have to be a part of everyone's diet. After all, there are countless healthy vegetarians in the world. For meat eaters, we suggest eating lean meat three times a week, plus eggs or skinless chicken once or twice a week, accompanied by plenty of salad and vegetables.
- Smaller eaters: 1–2 serves a day
- Medium eaters: 2–3 serves a day
- Bigger eaters: 3 serves a day

Dairy foods – what's a serve?

One serve is equivalent to:
- 1 cup (250 ml) low fat milk
- 1 cup (250 ml) calcium-enriched low fat soy milk
- 200 g tub low fat yoghurt or calcium-enriched soy yoghurt
- 40 g or two slices reduced-fat hard cheese such as cheddar
- 1 cup (250 ml) low fat custard is a calcium-equivalent option but is higher in kilojoules, so don't rely on it routinely.

How much a day?

Everyone should aim to eat or drink at least three serves of dairy foods or calcium-enriched soy products per day to meet their calcium needs. Post-menopausal women need 3–4 serves each day due to increased calcium needs.
- Smaller eaters: 3 serves
- Medium eaters: 3 serves
- Bigger eaters: 3–4 serves

INCLUDING LEAN MEATS AND LOW FAT DAIRY IN YOUR DIET
Breakfast
- Try poached or scrambled eggs on toast or an omelette.
- Fruit smoothies make a great breakfast when you are on the go.
- Yoghurt is a tasty accompaniment to muesli or fruit salad.

Lunch
- Gluten-free sandwiches and rolls can be filled with chicken and avocado; lean roast beef and mustard; turkey and cranberry sauce; sliced lamb with hommous; egg and lettuce; or lean ham and salad.

- If you prefer toasted sandwiches (a better choice when using most gluten-free breads), try chicken and avocado; ham, cheese and tomato; or ricotta, sundried tomato and rocket.
- Dress up your salad with lean roast meat, sliced chicken breast (no skin), a boiled egg or some cubes of low fat feta.
- Frittata made with eggs, low fat milk, chopped vegetables, lean ham, fresh herbs and low fat cheese make a tasty weekend lunch or brunch served with salad.
- Soups are a great winter warmer – try chicken and sweetcorn, beef and vegetable, or pea and ham.
- For a variation on your usual sandwich, try a gluten-free wrap filled with hommous, buckwheat tabbouli and sliced chicken breast or roast lamb.

Dinner

- Go for lean meats – marinate and grill or pan-fry with a little olive or canola oil.
- Beef and chicken can be sliced into strips and stir-fried with vegetables.
- For the barbecue, choose lean steak, marinated chicken breast or kebabs.
- Use lean meats in curries and casseroles. If you have time, cook the meal the day before, refrigerate and then skim fat from the top the next day before reheating to serve.
- Low fat yoghurt and ricotta mixed with chives make a low fat alternative to sour cream on vegetables or Mexican food.

Snacks and desserts

- Fruit smoothies or low fat milkshakes make a satisfying calcium-packed snack.
- Yoghurt is always a quick and easy option.
- Try a glass of gluten-free hot chocolate to satisfy those chocolate cravings.
- Ricotta can be used as a topping on gluten-free crackers or a spread on fruit loaf.
- For dessert, add a spoonful of low fat custard, frozen yoghurt or ice-cream to fruit.
- Low fat ricotta can also be used in cheesecakes or as a topping for fresh fruit.
- Low fat buttermilk can be used in baking and desserts.

Why do I never see a GI value for meat or cheese?

The foods we eat contain three main macro-nutrients – protein, carbohydrate and fat. Some foods, such as meat, are high in protein, while bread is high in carbohydrate and butter is high in fat. It is necessary for us to consume a variety of foods (in varying proportions) to provide all three nutrients, but the GI applies only to carbohydrate-containing foods. It is impossible for us to measure a GI value for foods that contain negligible carbohydrate. These foods include meat, fish, chicken, eggs, cheese, nuts, oil, cream and butter. There are other nutritional aspects you should consider when choosing these foods, such as the amount and type of fats they contain.

6. Eat more fish and seafood

Fish, particularly oily fish, is the best source of long-chain omega-3 fatty acids – fats that offer valuable health benefits. Long-chain omega-3s can help reduce blood clotting and inflammatory reactions, and studies have shown a link between regular fish consumption and a reduced risk of coronary heart disease. In fact, just one serving of fish a week may reduce the risk of a fatal heart attack by 40 per cent. Our bodies only make small amounts of these fatty acids, and so we rely on dietary sources, especially fish and seafood, for them. You should try to eat fish at least twice a week. Fresh fish that contains the highest amounts of omega-3 fats include:

- Swordfish
- Atlantic salmon
- Southern bluefin tuna
- Gemfish
- Silver perch, and
- Atlantic, Pacific and Spanish mackerel (blue mackerel).

Canned fish can also provide omega-3 fats, good sources being:

- Mackerel
- Salmon
- Sardines, and
- Tuna.

Try to choose varieties canned in spring water where possible. If you choose fish canned in oil, opt for those in olive or canola oil.

Just remember not to eat fish cooked in solid (saturated) fat. That means avoiding fried fish from fast-food restaurants, even if they say it's cooked in vegetable oil.

Fish and seafood – what's a serve?
One serve is equivalent to:
- 150 g raw fish or seafood
- 120 g grilled or steamed fish
- 100 g canned fish (drained)

How much a week?
Eat fish – including fresh, frozen, canned and smoked – at least twice a week, as an alternative to a serve of meat, chicken or eggs.

TIPS TO HELP YOU INCREASE YOUR INTAKE OF FISH
Breakfast
- Sardines on toast are filling and will give you a good dose of omega-3s.
- Try an omelette with smoked salmon or trout.

Lunch
- Add tuna or salmon to a gluten-free sandwich or salad.
- For something different, add salmon or tuna rissoles to a gluten-free roll with lettuce and avocado.
- Grilled fish with salad makes a healthy lunch choice when eating out.

Dinner
- Homemade fish and chips is a quick and easy meal to prepare. Wrap fish in foil with lemon juice and herbs and

bake in the oven. Make sweet potato chips by slicing and brushing or spraying with olive oil, and baking on a tray in the oven. Serve with salad or steamed vegetables.
- Try adding tuna, salmon or a seafood mix to gluten-free pasta with a tomato sauce and some vegetables.
- Barbecued fish makes a healthy alternative to sausages and fatty meats.
- Use fresh salmon in a stir-fry as it holds its shape.

7. Opt for monounsaturated and omega-3 polyunsaturated fats and oils such as olive, peanut and canola oils

It is not necessary, or beneficial, to cut all fats out of your diet. In fact, some fat is essential for your health, as it provides essential fatty acids and carries fat-soluble vitamins and antioxidants. So it's fine to use small amounts of oil in cooking and salad dressings, but it is important to choose the right ones. If you don't use oil, you can still get these 'good' fats by eating nuts, seeds, avocado, olives and fish.

While it is generally recommended that you replace saturated fats with either polyunsaturated or monounsaturated fats, there is something else to keep in mind. Omega-3 fats are one type of polyunsaturated fat (found mainly in oily fish but also in some plant foods including linseeds, flaxseed oil, walnuts, canola oil and soy products) which we know have many health benefits. But to make good use of the omega-3 fats in your diet it is important that you don't have too many omega-6 fats (the other type of polyunsaturated fat) – the ratio between them is important. Most people have too much omega-6 (found in most vegetable oils and margarines including sunflower, safflower and grapeseed as well as most nuts and seeds) and too little omega-3.

To improve this balance we recommend having a regular source of omega-3 fats in your diet and cooking most of the time with monounsaturated oils rather than the polyunsaturated variety. These include:

Olive oil which is high in monounsaturated fats and low in saturates with a minimal polyunsaturated fat content. This is an advantage, as it allows our bodies to make greater use of the omega-3 fats we obtain from other dietary sources, without any competition from excessive polyunsaturated omega-6 fats. Olive oil is also rich in antioxidants, which have many health benefits. Olive oil can be used in cooking and is a good choice for salad dressings. Olive oil margarines are also available.

Peanut oil which is a mild-tasting oil that oxidises slowly and can withstand high cooking temperatures. About 50 per cent of the fat in peanut oil is monounsaturated and another 30 per cent is polyunsaturated. This heart-healthy fat is suitable for Asian cooking such as stir-fries.

Canola oil which contains significant amounts of omega-3 fat, besides being high in monounsaturated fat. It's a multipurpose cooking oil and can also be used for baking cakes and muffins. Margarine made from canola oil is also available.

Flaxseed (linseed) oil which is the richest plant source of omega-3s and contains very little omega-6 fat. However, it is highly prone to oxidation (meaning the fats it contains turn rancid easily), so it shouldn't be heated and needs to be stored carefully. It is best used in salad dressings. Alternatively, flaxseeds (linseeds) can be freshly ground and sprinkled on cereals or added to cakes and muffins.

> ## What fat is that?
>
> Although foods contain a mixture of fatty acids, one type tends to predominate, allowing us to categorise foods according to their main fatty acid component. The asterisk (*) beside the foods listed below means the food is a good source of omega-3 fatty acids.
>
> **Polyunsaturated products**
> **Oils** – Safflower, sunflower, grapeseed, soy bean*, corn, linseed* (flaxseed), cottonseed, walnut*, sesame, evening primrose oils
> **Spreads** – polyunsaturated margarines, tahini (sesame seed paste)
> **Nuts and seeds** – walnuts*, sunflower seeds, pepitas (pumpkin seeds), sesame seeds
> **Other plant sources** – soy beans, soy milk, whole grains
> **Animal sources** – oily fish*
>
> **Monounsaturated products**
> **Oils** – olive, canola*, peanut, Sunola™, macadamia and mustard seed oils
> **Spreads** – olive oil margarines, canola margarine*, peanut butter
> **Nuts and seeds** – cashews, macadamias, almonds, hazelnuts, pecans, pistachio, peanuts
> **Other plant sources** – avocado, olives
> **Animal sources** – very lean red meat, lean chicken, lean pork, egg yolks

> **Saturated products**
> **Oils/fats** – palm and palm kernel oil, coconut oil, drippings, lard, copha, ghee, solid frying oils, cooking margarines and shortening
> **Spreads** – butter, cream cheese
> **Dairy foods** – full-fat dairy products: cheese, cream, sour cream, yoghurt, whole milk, ice-cream
> **Animal sources** – fat on beef and lamb, skin on chicken, sausage, salami, most luncheon meats

What to drink?

An adequate fluid intake is essential for good health, but most people don't drink enough. Most adults need about 2 litres of fluid each day (about 8 glasses) to replace the fluid that is lost from the body. More is needed in hot weather, during exercise, or if you work in air conditioning. An adequate fluid intake is important for kidney function, temperature regulation and for preventing constipation.

Water is the best fluid to quench your thirst and is also the best choice if you are watching your weight and blood glucose or insulin levels. Soft drinks, energy drinks and cordials contain large amounts of added sugar and it is best to avoid these where possible. Most fruit juices have a relatively low GI and can be consumed in moderation, but remember that they still contain a lot of carbohydrate from the natural fruit sugars. It would be better to eat the whole fruit (which still contains the fibre) rather than drinking the juice.

If you struggle to drink plain water, you could try mineral or soda water with a slice of lemon or lime and a few fresh mint leaves. Or try diluting fruit juice with water, soda water or mineral water. Tea is also acceptable. Green tea, in particular, has been shown to be high in antioxidants and may have many health benefits. If you like hot drinks, there are also a wide variety of herbal teas available, but if you are pregnant you need to be careful as some types are not suitable during pregnancy – check the label.

Coffee and alcohol have a diuretic effect, so should not be counted as part of your 8 glasses. Both are best consumed in moderation. Alcohol is also high in kilojoules so it should be limited when watching your weight. The recommendations are 2–3 standard drinks per day for men and 1–2 for women, with a few alcohol-free days per week. Beer contains gluten and should be avoided on a gluten-free diet although some gluten-free varieties are now available.

Milk and soy milk are low GI, and the low fat varieties are the best choice for adults and older children. Full-fat varieties should be given to children up to 2 years of age. If you don't like the taste of milk or soy milk on their own, you could add a teaspoon of gluten-free drinking chocolate for flavour, or make a fruit smoothie for a satisfying snack or breakfast on the run.

This for that

The bread and cereal group is where most of your decisions about GI need to be made. You may feel like your food choices are already restricted within this food group. But there are plenty of options available and changing to a low GI way of eating is often just a matter of swapping one food for another, as shown in the following table. You may actually find that you get more variety in your diet by choosing low GI.

SUBSTITUTING LOW GI FOR HIGH GI FOODS

High GI food	Low GI alternative
Bread – most gluten-free varieties	Choose those with whole kernel grains and/or legume flours (such as chickpea or soy flour) psyllium husks and those labelled as 'low GI'
Processed breakfast cereals made from puffed or flaked corn and rice	Gluten-free cereals containing rice bran and psyllium
Rice porridge	Quinoa porridge
Corn and rice crackers and crispbreads	Raw nut and seed mixes, roasted chickpeas or soy beans (chicknuts or soynuts), hommous dip with vegetable crudités
Gluten-free cakes and muffins	Make these with fruit, dried fruits, nuts, seeds, psyllium husks or rice bran
Potato	Carisma, Almera, baby chat potatoes, Nicola potatoes, orange sweet potato, sweetcorn, taro, yam and chestnuts
Rice	Longer grain varieties such as basmati, SunRice Doongara CleverRice™ or Moolgiri medium grain rice, or try Asian rice noodles
Gluten-free pasta	Lower GI varieties if available, or Asian rice noodles/vermicelli, buckwheat (soba) noodles or mung bean (bean thread) noodles

Low GI gluten-free baking

Q: *I'm a very keen cook. If I make my own gluten-free bread (or dumplings, pancakes, muffins etc), which flours, if any, are gluten-free and low GI?*

A: To date there are no GI ratings for refined flour whether it's made from rice, legumes or other gluten-free grains. This is because the GI rating of a food must be tested physiologically, that is in real people. So far we haven't had volunteers willing to tuck into 50 gram portions of flour on three occasions! What we do know, however, is that bakery products such as bread, cakes, biscuits and muffins made from refined flour, whether it's from rice, maize, buckwheat or other grains, are quickly digested and absorbed.

What should you do with your own baking? Try to increase the soluble fibre content by partially substituting rice or maize flour with legume flours (such as soy or chickpea flour – also known as besan) and increase the bulkiness of the product with dried fruit, nuts, seeds and psyllium husks. Don't think of it as a challenge. It's an opportunity for some creative cooking.

What to choose when eating out

Eating out on a gluten-free diet can be difficult, particularly as there is often gluten in items such as sauces, stock, dressings and gravy. It is important that the restaurant understands your need for a meal that is completely free of gluten and it may be a good idea to call beforehand to ensure that they can accommodate your needs.

Your state coeliac society should be able to give you a list of recommended restaurants to eat at, where you can be confident that they are able to provide you with a gluten-free meal. These are good places to start. Otherwise you need to ask plenty of questions and remember that, if you are in doubt, you are best to leave it out!

Following are some tips to making low GI gluten-free meal choices when eating out. It will vary from restaurant to restaurant, and it is always important to ask questions.

- Plain grilled steak, chicken or fish with a cob of sweetcorn, and salad or steamed vegetables.
- Indian dahl with basmati rice.
- Mexican tacos (if 100 per cent corn) with beans, salad, avocado, salsa and grated cheese.
- Sushi filled with raw fish or avocado and cucumber (no soy sauce).
- Vietnamese rice paper rolls (but hold the dipping sauce unless you can check if it is gluten-free).
- Asian rice noodles stir-fried with vegetables, tofu or prawns, peanuts, coriander and lemon or lime juice (check the sauces).
- Mixed-bean, chickpea or lentil salads (leave the dressing unless you can check it is gluten-free).
- Falafel (check they are gluten-free) with hommous and salad.

Chapter 6

Putting the GI to work in your day

This chapter contains four healthy 7-day menus for adults, adult vegetarians, teens and schoolchildren with an emphasis on low GI carbs, lean protein, plenty of fruit and vegetables, and the good oils. We have included recipes from the book (marked with an asterisk) to inspire you to try the recipes in Part 3.

The adult menus don't include snacks, but we have suggested some for teenagers and schoolchildren. The teenagers' and children's menus also reflect different taste preferences and energy needs during this vital time of growth and development.

7-day Menu – Adult

	Monday	Tuesday	Wednesday
Breakfast	Creamy Muesli with Berries*	Wholegrain gluten-free toast with baked beans	Peachy Pistachio Porridge*
Lunch	Individual Spanish Tortilla* with salad Fresh fruit	Gluten-free wrap with chicken breast, avocado and salad Fresh fruit	Chicken Pasta Salad with Mango Salsa* Dried fruit and nut mix
Dinner	Barbecued Lemon Chicken Skewers with Bean and Asparagus Pilaf* Fruit yoghurt	Salmon and Pumpkin Patties with Butter Bean Salad* Garden salad Low fat gluten-free hot chocolate	Greek-style Beef Skewers* Fresh fruit salad with yoghurt

Thursday	Friday	Saturday	Sunday
Turkey, Avocado and Fresh Peach Salsa Wrap*	Seriously Strawberry Smoothie*	Breakfast Fried Rice*	Gluten-free toast with scrambled eggs and grilled tomato
Velvety Pumpkin, Soup* Fresh fruit	Warm Potato Salad with Herbs and Toasted Hazelnuts* Fresh fruit	Tuna Pasta Niçoise* Fruit yoghurt	Thai Beef Salad with Chilli Lime Dressing* Fresh fruit
Lamb Curry with Spinach Rice Pilaf* Berry Yoghurt Delight*	Pork, Bok Choy and Noodle Stir-Fry* Low fat gluten-free hot chocolate	Cranberry Chicken with Quinoa* Green beans and carrots Berry and Pear Cobbler*	Herb Fish Parcels with Fennel, Bean and Tomato Salad* Rhubarb and Apple Crumble* with fat-reduced gluten-free custard

7-day Menu – Adult Vegetarian

	Monday	Tuesday	Wednesday
Breakfast	Gluten-free Granola with Pecans and Almonds* with low fat milk or gluten-free soy milk	Wholegrain gluten-free toast with baked beans	Peachy Pistachio Porridge*
Lunch	Carrot, Avocado and Snow Pea Rice Paper Rolls* Fresh fruit	Chunky Tomato Soup with Chickpeas* Dried fruit and nut mix	Warm Potato Salad with Herbs and Toasted Hazelnuts* Fresh fruit
Dinner	Vegetarian Pad Thai* Fruit yoghurt	Spinach Rice Pilaf* (see Lamb Curry with Spinach Pilaf) with pine nuts Gluten-free hot chocolate	Tofu Laksa* (see Prawn Laksa – variation) Cranberry Baked Apple* with low fat yoghurt

Note: Choose soy products (milk, custard, yoghurt) fortified with vitamin B_{12} where possible, or take a vitamin B_{12} supplement

Thursday	Friday	Saturday	Sunday
Wholegrain gluten-free toast with avocado and tomato	Banana and Passionfruit Smoothie*	Multigrain Porridge with Apple*	Tofu Hotcakes with Avocado, Tomato and Corn Salsa*
Avocado and Tofu Sushi* Fresh fruit	Gluten-free pasta salad tossed with roasted butternut pumpkin, chickpeas and pine nuts Fresh fruit	Lentil and Feta Salad* Dried fruit and nut mix	Velvety Pumpkin, Soup* Fresh fruit
Pumpkin, Ricotta and Lentil Lasagne* Gluten-free hot chocolate	Tofu, Bok Choy and Rice Noodle Stir-Fry* (see Pork, Bok Choy and Rice Noodle Stir-Fry – variation) Fruit salad with low fat yoghurt	Falafel* with Pistachio and Quinoa Tabbouli*, and Hommous* Chocolate Almond Cake* with reduced-fat gluten-free custard	Chilli Bean Tacos* (see Chicken Taco – variation) Rhubarb and Apple Crumble* with fat reduced gluten-free custard

7-day Menu – Teenager

	Monday	Tuesday	Wednesday
Breakfast	Multigrain Porridge with Apple* Glass of fruit juice SNACK: Dried fruit and nut mix and a banana	Ricotta, Strawberry and Banana Wrap* Glass of milk SNACK: Apple plus gluten-free crackers and cheese	Creamy Muesli with Berries* SNACK: Apple and Pecan Muffin*
Lunch	Gluten-free wrap with turkey, avocado and salad Fresh fruit SNACK: Fruit yoghurt	Chicken Pasta Salad with Mango Salsa* Fresh fruit SNACK: Fruit Loaf* with gluten-free hot chocolate	Individual Spanish Tortilla* SNACK: Gluten-free toast with peanut butter
Dinner	Salmon and Pumpkin Patties* with peas and beans Chocolate Mousse*	Homemade gluten-free pizza Berry Pear Cobbler*	Chicken Tacos* Fruit salad with yoghurt

Thursday	Friday	Saturday	Sunday
Wholegrain gluten-free toast with peanut butter Gluten-free hot chocolate SNACK: Banana plus Apricot Nut slice*	Banana and Passionfruit Smoothie* SNACK: Rice cakes with peanut butter	Apricot and Strawberry Parfait Crunch* SNACK: Apple plus dried fruit and nut mix	Wholegrain gluten-free toasted sandwich with baked beans and cheese SNACK: Apple
Easy Tuna Bake* with cherry tomatoes Dried fruit and nut mix SNACK: Fruit yoghurt	Sushi with Salmon* SNACK: Muesli Nut Biscuit* plus a glass of milk	Chicken Nuggets with Salad* Fresh fruit SNACK: Fruit smoothie	Rice Paper Rolls* SNACK: Cheese and gluten-free crackers
Pork, Bok Choy and Rice Noodle Stir-Fry* Gluten-free hot chocolate	Pasta with Italian Meatballs in Tomato Sauce* and salad Rhubarb and Apple Crumble* with reduced-fat ice cream	Thai Beef Salad with Chilli Lime Dressing* Passionfruit Banana Cups with Lime Coconut Macaroons*	Beef and Bean Fajitas* Berry Yoghurt Delight*

7-day Menu – Schoolchild

	Monday	Tuesday	Wednesday
Breakfast	Fresh fruit combo with yoghurt SNACK: Small box of sultanas	Ricotta, Strawberry and Banana Wrap* SNACK: Apple	Gluten-free cereal with milk and sliced peaches SNACK: Handful of dried fruit
Lunch	Gluten-free wrap with ham cheese and pineapple Fruit salad SNACK: Fruit yoghurt	Rice Paper Rolls* SNACK: Fruit Loaf* with gluten-free hot chocolate	Chicken Nuggets with Salad* SNACK: Gluten-free toast with peanut butter
Dinner	Easy Chicken and Corn Soup* with gluten-free toast Berry Yoghurt Delight* (served in a parfait glass)	Shepherds pie with carrots and peas Banana split	Homemade fried rice Yoghurt Strawberry Jelly*

Thursday	Friday	Saturday	Sunday
Wholegrain gluten-free toast with baked beans SNACK: Grapes	Seriously Strawberry Smoothie* SNACK: Gluten-free crackers with peanut butter	Breakfast Fried Rice* SNACK: Orange	Gluten-free toast with scrambled egg SNACK: Apple
Individual Spanish Tortilla* Box of sultanas SNACK: Fruit pieces with yoghurt dip	Gluten-free wrap with peanut butter, sultanas and grated carrot Kiwi fruit SNACK: Brownie*	Baked Bean gluten-free wholegrain toasted sandwich SNACK: Sultanas and glass of milk	Gluten-free homemade pizza SNACK: Banana and Passionfruit Smoothie*
Chicken Tacos* Chocolate Mousse*	Easy Tuna Bake* with salad Rhubarb and Apple Crumble* with ice-cream	Chicken and Rice Lettuce Cups* Passionfruit Banana Cups* with Lime and Coconut Macaroons*	Spaghetti with Italian Meatballs in Tomato Sauce* Frozen fruit kebabs

Part 3

Eat yourself healthy

Recipes with a healthy balance for breakfast, lunch, dinner, desserts and snacks. Plus plenty of options for the school lunchbox.

Cooking the low GI way

One of the aims of our books is to show you easy ways to lower the GI of your diet. For those who like to cook, low (or lower) GI recipes are part of the picture. Even if you don't like the following recipes, you will find that they give you ideas of how you can use low GI ingredients in flavourful and nutritious combinations.

Naturally we aim to develop recipes with as low a GI as possible and most of the recipes in this book are low GI, but there are a few popular dishes for which even we find this difficult! Typically these are baked goods made with flour such as muffins and cakes. Because flour is a finely milled product, it is rapidly digested and has a high GI. By incorporating lower GI carbs and lots of fibre such as whole kernel grains, rice bran, psyllium husks, fruit, milk and juices into these recipes we can lower the GI.

Modern diets contain much more sodium (salt) than is commensurate with good health, so one of our guidelines when creating recipes is to limit sodium intake. We don't add salt to our cooking and we use salt-reduced gluten-free products where possible. You may think cutting salt will be difficult but your tastebuds will adapt pretty quickly. You can add flavour to your meals by using herbs and spices, lemon juice and pepper. You may like to invest in a good pepper grinder!

NUTRIENT PROFILE

Each recipe is accompanied by a nutrient profile* which gives you a snapshot of its key nutritional attributes. The profile normally relates to a single serve, assuming you divide the

---

* Recipes have been analysed using nutrient analysis software, FoodWorks(®) (Xyris Software) based on Australian and New Zealand food composition data.

recipe to make the specified number of serves, or to one item for wraps, tacos, fajitas, muffins, biscuits etc. If you eat a double or triple serve of the recipe, then you would scale up the figures two or three times respectively.

In the nutrient profile for the recipes we include kilojoules, fat (including saturated fat), fibre, protein and carbohydrate.

Kilojoules

The smaller the number, the fewer the kilojoules (or fuel) in a serve. This is a good thing if you have a tendency to gain weight. By incorporating lots of vegetables, salads, fruits and whole kernel grains into the recipes, we have ensured that many have a low energy density. This means that they are bulky and filling without providing lots of kilojoules.

Fat

The fat content is given in grams per serve (or item). This is useful if you are trying to eat a low fat diet. If the figure seems a little high on some recipes, rest assured it is mostly 'good' fat or of a poly- or monounsaturated nature. A low saturated fat intake is recommended for everyone and all our recipes are low in saturated fat.

Fibre

Experts recommend a daily fibre intake of 30 grams, but most people fall short of that, averaging 20–25 grams. And it can be more difficult to get enough fibre on a gluten-free diet due to the absence of many grain foods. You'll find that most of our recipes are fibre-rich. This means they'll not only keep you regular but will help lower your blood glucose, your cholesterol levels and reduce your risk of many chronic diseases.

Protein

The protein content is given in grams per serve. Most of us get plenty of protein without having to think about it. Sufficient protein in the diet is important for weight control because compared with carbohydrate and fat, protein makes us feel more satisfied immediately after eating and reduces hunger between meals. Protein also increases our metabolic rate for 1–3 hours after eating. This means we burn more energy by the minute compared with the increase that occurs after eating carbohydrates or fats. Even though this is a relatively small difference it may be important in long-term weight control.

Carbohydrate

The amount of carbohydrate per serve in grams may be of most interest to those with diabetes. Because the GI only relates to the carbohydrate content of foods, you will find that most of our recipes have a significant carbohydrate content.

MEASURES

¼ teaspoon	=	1.25 ml
½ teaspoon	=	2.5 ml
1 teaspoon	=	5 ml
1 tablespoon	=	20 ml
¼ cup	=	60 ml
⅓ cup	=	80 ml
½ cup	=	125 ml
⅔ cup	=	160 ml
¾ cup	=	190 ml
1 cup	=	250 ml
2 cups	=	500 ml

INGREDIENTS

Breadcrumbs

To make fresh gluten-free breadcrumbs:

Tear slices of gluten-free bread, including the crusts, into 3 or 4 pieces and process in a food processor. It's a good idea to make extra breadcrumbs while you have the processor running and freeze the rest in 1-cup quantities. They will defrost very quickly when you need to use them.

Store in an airtight plastic container (a zip-lock bag would be fine) in the freezer for up to 2 months.

- 1 slice Country Life Low GI Gluten Free bread makes about ⅓ cup. If you don't have a food processor, grate bread using a coarse grater.

To make dried gluten-free breadcrumbs:

Preheat the oven to 180°C. Cut the bread into 4 squares. Lay squares on a wire rack and place in a baking dish. Bake for 10–15 minutes or until just coloured. Turn off the oven and leave bread there for 20–25 minutes or until bread is hard. Break the bread into smaller pieces and process in a food processor until crumbed.

- 2 slices of Country Life Low GI Gluten Free bread makes about ½ cup dried breadcrumbs. If you don't have a food processor, put the bread in a strong plastic bag and crush with a rolling pin.

Eggs

We use 59 gram eggs in our recipes.

Flour

In our recipes we use a variety of different gluten-free flours including rice flour, brown rice flour, besan (chickpea flour), buckwheat flour, cornflour and potato flour. You'll find these in larger supermarkets and health food stores. When buying cornflour, make sure you get the gluten-free variety (made from corn) as regular cornflour is not actually corn but fine wheat flour. Make sure you buy gluten-free baking powder, too.

Margarine

We use reduce-fat poly- or monounsaturated fat margarines in our cooking.

Pasta

As we explained earlier, many gluten-free pastas made from rice or corn have a high GI. That's why we combine pasta with lots of low GI ingredients in our recipes. Soy pastas may be lower GI than those made from corn or rice flour.

Potatoes

We use the low GI (55) Carisma potatoes in our recipes. They have a creamy yellow skin with yellow flesh, and a firm, waxy cooked texture, and are ideal for steaming and boiling, and in salads. Rinse them thoroughly in cold water and scrub before cooking. Take care not to overcook them or they will absorb too much water. If you have trouble finding these (they are currently available exclusively in Coles supermarkets),

Nicola, Almera or baby new ('chat') potatoes are the next best choices, having a lower GI than other varieties of potato.

Rice

We use the lower GI rices in our recipes and as serving suggestions – basmati (GI 58), SunRice Doongara CleverRice™ (GI 54) and Moolgiri medium grain rice (GI 54).

Spices

A number of recipes have pre-mixed herb and spice blends. We like the Herbie's brand because the quality and flavour are outstanding and, aside from asafoetida and blends containing asafoetida, they are all gluten-free. Check all labels on supermarket brands carefully for gluten content and if you're unsure, see page 248 for more information on how to buy the Herbie's range. Always check the labels when buying spice blends as some may contain gluten.

Spring onions or shallots?

This is very much 'what's in a name'. Australians have traditionally used the term 'shallot' for what is technically a scallion, spring onion or green onion. The word 'shallot' comes from the French 'eschalote', referring to a small, papery-skinned onion that looks like garlic. In this book we use the term 'spring onion'.

Stock

If you don't have time to make your own stock, check that the one you buy is gluten-free and reduced-salt. Massel is a good brand to look for and is widely available in supermarkets.

Tamari

You can buy tamari from Asian produce stores and the Asian section of supermarkets. Gluten-free tamari is one of the authentic soy sauce recipes first introduced to Japan from China. It is a wheat-free sauce made from soy beans and has a slightly stronger flavour than regular soy sauce. It's traditionally used to flavour longer cooking foods (soups, stews etc), but it can be used in marinades and dressings too, or as a condiment or dipping sauce. Look for reduced-salt tamari.

Xanthan gum

You'll find this handy ingredient in health food stores or the health food aisle of major supermarkets. It's widely used in gluten-free baking to improve the texture of the final product. It's more expensive than baking powder, but a small sachet goes a long way.

Chapter 7: Breakfasts and brunches

A healthy breakfast that includes gluten-free wholegrains and fruit is a great start in meeting your daily fibre intake. Nourish your body, recharge your brain, boost your metabolism and power your day with our tasty breakfasts and brunches.

GI Express: breakfast basics

HOT!
Cereal plus
Start with a bowl of steaming quinoa porridge (made with whole grains, not flakes). Add lots of fresh or frozen berries, stirring them in gently. Top with a dollop of low fat natural yoghurt and a sprinkling of sugar.

Toast plus
Start by toasting a low GI gluten-free bread such as Country Life Low GI Gluten Free bread (GI 53). Add 2–3 tablespoons of creamed corn and spread it over evenly. Top with fresh

mushroom slices, a slice or two of tomato and a sprinkle of light mozzarella cheese. Grill until the cheese melts and the corn is bubbly.

COLD!
Cereal plus
Start with your favourite gluten-free muesli, a low GI one like Freedom Foods Gluten Free, Wheat Free Muesli with psyllium (GI 50) is a good choice. Add low fat milk and fresh slices of apple or pear; ½ cup sliced strawberries, blueberries, or orange segments; or ½ banana, sliced. Top with a dollop of natural or flavoured low fat yoghurt and a sprinkle of chopped nuts.

Toast plus
Start by toasting a low GI gluten-free bread such as Country Life Low GI Gluten Free bread. Add 2–3 tablespoons of fresh ricotta and spread it over evenly. Top with a dollop of all-fruit spread such as apricot or strawberry, or a drizzle of pure floral honey.

Creamy Muesli with Berries

This recipe makes a thick muesli. If you prefer a 'runnier' texture, add extra milk before serving. The textures of brown rice flakes vary considerably between brands. Some are actually a breakfast-cereal flake like corn flakes. Look for smaller, denser, heavier flakes to use as an ingredient. The brand we used in our cooking (Four Leaf Organic) weighed in at 50 grams per half cup.

Serves 1 **Soaking time** Overnight **Preparation time** 5 minutes

⅓ cup (35 g) brown rice flakes
2 teaspoons rice bran
⅓ cup (80 ml) low fat milk or soy milk
½ apple, grated with skin on
1 teaspoon psyllium husks

To serve

¼ cup blueberries or sliced strawberries
1 tablespoon low fat natural yoghurt or soy yoghurt
1 tablespoon slivered almonds, lightly toasted

1. The night before, place the rice flakes, rice bran and milk in a bowl. Cover and leave in the refrigerator overnight.

2. In the morning, stir in the grated apple and psyllium husks and top with berries, a dollop or two of yoghurt and the slivered, toasted almonds.

VARIATIONS

- Replace the milk with orange juice.
- Replace the almonds with chopped walnuts – they don't need toasting.
- Replace the berries with your favourite fruit such as ½ banana, sliced; pulp of 1–2 passionfruit; canned (in water or natural juice) peach or pear slices, apricot halves or 1–2 plums.

PER SERVE

1295 kJ; 8 g fat (including 1.5 g saturated fat); 7 g fibre; 10 g protein; 45 g carbohydrate

Gluten-free Granola with Pecans and Almonds

It doesn't quite snap, crackle and pop – but it comes pretty close. The secret is in the slow cooking. You don't have to worry about it burning as it gently toasts to a golden brown in a low oven. After you have made it a couple of times, mix and match the ingredients to suit your family's likes and dislikes. The granola can be stored in a cool cupboard for up to ten days.

Makes about 8 cups **Preparation time** 15 minutes **Cooking time** 30 minutes

- 1 cup (15 g) brown puffed rice
- 1 cup (10 g) puffed buckwheat
- 1 cup (15 g) puffed millet
- ½ cup (50 g) quinoa flakes
- ½ cup (50 g) brown rice flakes
- 3 tablespoons rice bran
- 1 cup (130 g) roughly chopped pecan nuts
- 1 cup (80 g) slivered almonds
- ½ cup (60 g) pepitas (pumpkin seeds)
- ½ cup sunflower seeds
- 2 tablespoons (40 ml) walnut or canola oil
- ¼ cup (60 ml) pure floral honey
- 1 cup craisins (or sultanas or currants)

1. Preheat the oven to 150°C.
2. To make the granola, combine the grains, nuts and seeds in a large bowl and mix together well.
3. In a small saucepan, blend the oil and honey, and cook over a low heat until it is just melted. Set aside.
4. Stir the syrup mixture into the bowl of granola until the ingredients are lightly coated.
5. Spread evenly over a large, rimmed oven tray. Bake for 30 minutes, stirring halfway through to toast evenly, or until golden brown. Cool completely on the tray then add the dried fruit. Spoon into a large airtight container.
6. Serve ½ cup granola with ¼ cup milk and 1 tablespoon yoghurt.

VARIATIONS
- Add chopped dates, figs, quartered figlets or sliced apricots.
- For a tangy change, moisten with a little sour cherry or pomegranate juice.

PER SERVE INCLUDING MILK AND YOGHURT
1204 kJ; 17 g fat (including 2.0 g saturated fat); 3 g fibre; 9 g protein; 25 g carbohydrate

Banana and Passionfruit Smoothie

For a really delicious smoothie, the trick is to make sure the milk is very cold. Freeze leftovers for after-school ice blocks on hot days.

Serves 2 **Preparation time** 5 minutes

1 medium banana, chopped
1 cup (250 ml) low fat milk or light gluten-free soy milk, chilled
1 tub (200 g) low fat passionfruit yoghurt or gluten-free soy yoghurt
2 teaspoons rice bran
2 teaspoons pure floral honey (optional)

1 Combine all the ingredients in a blender and blend until smooth. Pour into two tall glasses and serve.

PER SERVE
900 kJ; 2 g fat (including 1.5 g saturated fat); 1.5 g fibre; 11 g protein; 36 g carbohydrate

Bananas

Bananas are not only fat-free and high in dietary fibre, they are a good source of carbohydrate for energy. They are also an excellent source of potassium and high in vitamin B6. Firm bananas have a low GI but this increases as they ripen, as some of the starches change into sugars.

Bananas make the ideal portable snack but can also be used in cakes, muffins, pancakes, smoothies and desserts such as puddings, soufflés and the good old banana split!

Custard Apple and Orange Smoothie

Custard apples are in season at the end of summer. The season is short so make the most of this creamy fruit that tastes like a tropical fruit salad and is a good source of carbs, protein, fibre and essential vitamins and minerals.

Serves 2 **Preparation time** 5 minutes

1 cup (250 ml) pulp custard apple
½ cup (125 ml) low fat milk or light gluten-free soy milk, chilled
½ cup (125 ml) orange juice
1 tub (200 g) low fat vanilla yoghurt or gluten-free soy yoghurt
2 teaspoons rice bran
2 teaspoons pure floral honey (optional)

1. Combine all the ingredients in a blender and blend until smooth. Pour into two tall glasses and serve.

PER SERVE
1085 kJ; 2.5 g fat (including 1 g saturated fat); 4 g fibre; 11 g protein; 47 g carbohydrate

Custard apples

Don't be put off by its green bumpy skin – a custard apple tastes rather like a tropical fruit salad all in one fruit! The ripe ones give slightly when you gently squeeze them, much like avocados. Simply cut in half and scoop out the white flesh. You can eat them raw, add to fruit salads or mashed bananas, make into ice-creams and sorbets, drinks, desserts, fillings for cakes and as an accompaniment to spicy dishes such as curry. Serve cut wedges on a fruit and cheese platter, but brush them with a little lemon juice first to prevent discolouring.

Seriously Strawberry Smoothie

You can make this with any berry-flavoured yoghurt – or with any mixture of berries for that matter.

Serves 2 **Preparation time** 5 minutes

1 punnet (200 g) strawberries, hulled
1 cup (250 ml) low fat milk or light gluten-free soy milk, chilled
1 tub (200 g) low fat strawberry yoghurt or gluten-free soy yoghurt
2 teaspoons rice bran
2 teaspoons pure floral honey (optional)

1 Combine all the ingredients in a blender and blend until smooth. Pour into two tall glasses and serve.

PER SERVE
809 kJ; 2 g fat (including 1.5 g saturated fat); 2.5 g fibre; 12 g protein; 29 g carbohydrate

Berries

Berries are a great source of folate, vitamin C and antioxidants which can protect the body against the effects of ageing and a range of degenerative diseases. Berries have also been shown to display anti-cancer properties, and cranberries can help reduce the risk of urinary tract infections. Versatile and with natural sweetness, berries can be eaten on their own, served with yoghurt or ice-cream, sliced on top of cereal, added to fruit salads, platters and cheese boards, used in mousses, tarts, muffins and cakes, or made into jam.

Apricot and Strawberry Parfait Crunch

Tempt those sleepy-heads and brekkie skippers with a parfait treat. We leave the skin on the apricots, but you can peel them (as you would peel tomatoes) if you prefer. In the cooler months, when fresh apricots aren't in season, it's delicious made with apricot compote (made with dried apricots) or even with canned (in water or natural juice) apricot halves. For the mixed nuts, choose from almonds, walnuts, pistachios, hazelnuts, Brazil nuts and cashews.

Serves 4 **Preparation time** 10 minutes **Cooking time** 1–2 minutes

⅓ cup (50 g) mixed raw nuts
3 tablespoons sunflower seeds
3 tablespoons pepitas (pumpkin seeds)
8 fresh apricots, washed
600 g low fat vanilla yoghurt
1 punnet (200 g) strawberries, sliced (or other berries in season)

1 Heat a non-stick frying pan over medium heat and add the nuts and seeds. Toast gently for 1–2 minutes, stirring continuously, or until just golden brown (take care, as nuts burn very quickly). Remove from the heat and spread nuts on a piece of kitchen paper. When cool enough to handle, chop roughly.

2 Halve the apricots, remove the stones and cut each half into 2–3 slices.

3 Take 4 tall glasses and spoon a little yoghurt into the bottom of each one. Divide the apricot slices among the glasses, top with another layer of yoghurt then finish with a layer of strawberries. Top with a good sprinkle of the crunchy toasted nut and seed mixture.

PER SERVE
1437 kJ; 15 g fat (including 1.5 g saturated fat); 6 g fibre; 16 g protein; 31 g carbohydrate

Peachy Pistachio Porridge

Peaches (poached or canned) and pistachios make a great combo with creamy quinoa porridge. Use peaches canned in water or natural juice.

Serves 4 **Preparation time** 10 minutes **Cooking time** 15 minutes

1 cup (200 g) quinoa, rinsed
2 cups (500 ml) low fat milk or gluten-free soy milk
1 apple, chopped with skin on
1 cinnamon stick or ½ teaspoon ground cinnamon
2 teaspoons psyllium husks

To serve

4 poached or canned peach halves
4 tablespoons low fat vanilla yoghurt
3 tablespoons finely chopped pistachios
1 cup low fat milk or gluten-free soy milk

1 Combine the rinsed quinoa with the milk in a saucepan. Bring to the boil over a medium heat (make sure that the milk doesn't boil over), then reduce the heat to low and simmer gently, stirring occasionally, for 5 minutes. Add the apple and cinnamon and simmer for 5–6 minutes, or until all liquid is absorbed and porridge is creamy. Remove the cinnamon stick, if using. Stir in the psyllium husks.

2 Spoon the porridge into breakfast bowls and serve topped with peach halves or slices, a tablespoon of yoghurt, a sprinkle of pistachios and a little milk.

VARIATIONS
- Try poached or canned plums for a tangy change.
- Chopped walnuts or lightly toasted almond slivers make a crunchy topping.

PER SERVE
1655 kJ; 9 g fat (including 2 g saturated fat); 7.5 g fibre; 17 g protein; 57 g carbohydrate

Multigrain Porridge with Apple

There's nothing better on a cold morning than a warming breakfast. Enjoy this combination of grains and nuts as is or, if you wish, add a tablespoon or two of sultanas for extra texture. We like using cloudy apple juice because research shows it has almost four times more antioxidants than clear juice. And it's naturally sweet so you don't need to top it with extra sugar or honey.

Serves 4 **Preparation time** 5 minutes **Cooking time** 5 minutes

⅓ cup (50 g) quinoa flakes
⅓ cup (50 g) brown rice flakes
½ teaspoon ground cinnamon
1 tablespoon rice bran
600 ml cloudy apple juice
2 teaspoons psyllium husks
¼ cup (40 g) finely chopped mixed nuts (almonds, cashews, Brazil nuts, macadamias, hazelnuts, walnuts)

To serve

1 cup (250 ml) low fat milk or gluten-free soy milk
4 tablespoons low fat plain or flavoured yoghurt (optional)

1. Place the quinoa flakes, rice flakes, cinnamon, rice bran and juice in a saucepan, and bring to the boil over a medium heat. Reduce the heat to low and simmer gently for 2–3 minutes, stirring occasionally, or until the liquid is absorbed and you have a creamy porridge.

2. Remove from heat and stir in the psyllium husks and finely chopped nuts. Spoon the porridge into breakfast bowls and serve with milk and a tablespoon of yoghurt.

PER SERVE
1109 kJ; 7 g fat (including 1.5 g saturated fat); 3.5 g fibre; 8 g protein; 42 g carbohydrate

Ricotta, Strawberry and Banana Wraps

Kate's favourite flatbread is Gluten Free Organic Tannour Bread – it's delicious but, sadly, not widely available. Look for it in organic or health food stores. There are a growing number of gluten-free flatbreads in supermarkets, but no published GI values for them yet. So, make sure your fillings include low GI ingredients.

Makes 2 **Preparation time** 5 minutes

100 g reduced-fat ricotta or cottage cheese
2 sheets gluten-free flatbread
1 medium banana, sliced
½ cup (60 g) finely sliced strawberries

1. Spread the ricotta over two-thirds of each flatbread and top with banana and strawberry slices. Wrap to enclose the filling and serve.

PER WRAP
1095 kJ; 7 g fat (including 3 g saturated fat); 2.5 g fibre; 8 g protein; 40 g carbohydrate

Turkey, Avocado and Fresh Peach Salsa Wraps

Makes 2 **Preparation time** 15 minutes

4 cos or iceberg lettuce leaves, roughly shredded
2 sheets gluten-free flatbread
4 gluten-free turkey slices
½ avocado, peeled, stone removed and finely sliced

Fresh Peach Salsa
1 peach, peeled and chopped
½ Lebanese cucumber, chopped
2 teaspoons chopped mint
1 spring onion, finely sliced

1. To make the salsa, combine all ingredients in a bowl. Set aside.

2. Spread the shredded lettuce over two-thirds of each flatbread and top each with 2 turkey slices and 2 avocado slices.

3. Spoon the Fresh Peach Salsa over the turkey and roll up to enclose the filling. If not serving immediately, wrap in paper or foil and store in the refrigerator for up to 5 hours.

VARIATION
- Replace the peach salsa with a tablespoon of cranberry jelly.

PER WRAP
1555 kJ; 18 g fat (including 3.5 g saturated fat); 3 g fibre; 17 g protein; 34 g carbohydrate

Breakfast Fried Rice

When preparing rice for evening meals, cook extra so you have leftovers. This fried rice is also a good one for the lunchbox. Look for tamari sauce in the Asian section of your supermarket.

Serves 4 **Preparation time** 5 minutes **Cooking time** 10 minutes

Ingredients:
- canola oil spray
- 2 eggs, at room temperature
- 3 teaspoons canola oil
- 1 small red capsicum, finely chopped
- 1 cup (150 g) frozen corn kernels, thawed
- 1 cup (150 g) frozen peas, thawed
- 3 cups (600 g) cooked basmati or Doongara Clever rice
- 3 spring onions, finely sliced on the diagonal
- 2 tablespoons reduced-salt gluten-free tamari
- ¼ cup lightly toasted and chopped cashews

1. Heat a large non-stick frying pan (or wok) over medium heat and spray with canola oil spray to coat the base (or sides of the wok). Whisk the eggs until frothy, pour into the pan and swirl to cover the base (or sides of the wok). Cook for 2 minutes or until the egg is set. Carefully loosen the edges, turn out onto a large plate and set aside to cool. Roll up the omelette, cut into thin strips and set aside.

2. Heat the canola oil in the pan over medium-high heat. Add the capsicum, corn and peas, and cook, tossing gently, for 2 minutes or until heated through. Add the rice and stir-fry for 2–3 minutes or until heated through. Add the sliced omelette, spring onions and tamari sauce, and stir-fry to heat through and combine well.

3. Serve topped with the toasted cashew nuts.

VARIATION
- Replace the corn, peas and capsicum with 3 cups frozen corn, peas and carrot mix.

PER SERVE
1631 kJ; 14 g fat (including 2 g saturated fat); 5.5 g fibre; 12 g protein; 51 g carbohydrate

Tofu Hotcakes with Avocado, Tomato and Corn Salsa

These hotcakes are also delicious served with oven-roasted tomatoes or sautéed mushrooms. Keep the cooked hotcakes warm on a plate covered with foil in a very low-heat oven, about 120°C, while cooking the remaining batter. Halve the quantities if you only want to make 4.

Makes 8 **Preparation time** 15 minutes **Cooking time** 40 minutes

300 g silken tofu, drained
2 eggs
1 cup (250 ml) low fat gluten-free soy milk
1 cup (150 g) rice flour
½ cup (125 g) besan (chickpea) flour
1 tablespoon gluten-free baking powder
canola oil spray

Avocado, Tomato and Corn Salsa
1 cob corn (or 1 cup (150 g) canned or frozen corn kernels)
2 ripe tomatoes, finely chopped
1 small ripe avocado, finely chopped
½ small red (Spanish) onion, finely chopped
1 small red chilli, finely chopped
⅓ cup finely chopped coriander
2 tablespoons fresh lime juice
1 tablespoon olive oil
freshly ground black pepper

1 Preheat oven to 120°C to keep the hotcakes warm once you have made them.

2 To make the salsa, microwave or steam the corn (if using fresh cob) until just tender. Set aside to cool slightly. Cut the kernels off the cob and place them in a bowl with the tomato, avocado, onion, chilli, coriander, lime juice and oil. Stir gently, season with pepper, and set aside.

3 To make the hotcakes, place the tofu in a bowl and use a fork to mash. Whisk in the eggs and soy milk. Sift the rice flour, besan and baking powder into a bowl, add to the tofu mixture and mix until well combined.

4 Spray a large non-stick frying pan with canola oil and place over a medium heat. Drop ⅓ cup (80 ml) of the batter into the pan and spread out to about a 10 cm diameter. Cook for 3 minutes or until golden underneath. Turn carefully and cook a further 2 minutes or until the hotcake has risen and is golden brown and cooked through. Repeat with the remaining batter to make 8 hotcakes.

5 To serve, place a hotcake on each plate and top with the salsa. Cover any leftover salsa and store in the refrigerator for up to 2 days.

VARIATIONS
- For a quicker and easier topping, replace the Avocado, Tomato and Corn Salsa with a 400 g can of baked beans combined with creamed corn.
- The salsa can also be replaced with oven-roasted tomatoes or sautéed mushrooms.

PER HOTCAKE
1406 kJ; 16 g fat (including 3 g saturated fat); 5 g fibre; 14 g protein; 32 g carbohydrate

10 toast-topper tips

Many gluten-free breads taste much better toasted. Here are some toppings and fillings that will help power your day.

- Baked beans topped with grated reduced-fat cheese
- Creamed corn topped with lean gluten-free ham
- Scrambled egg with basil
- Sautéed mushrooms with parsley
- Labne (yoghurt cheese) with cucumber and tomato slices
- Avocado, spinach and tomato slices
- Ricotta, sliced pears or apples and chopped walnuts
- Hommous and tomato
- Avocado with canned Mexi beans
- Ricotta, sliced plums and slivered almonds

Portobello Pizzas with Parmesan Crumb

This filling brunch will just about power you for the rest of the day. It's also great served as a light meal.

Serves 6 **Preparation time** 10 minutes **Cooking time** 30 minutes

2–3 tablespoons olive oil
6 portobello (or field) mushrooms, wiped, stems removed and chopped
1 onion, finely chopped
3 cloves garlic, finely chopped
1 small red capsicum, finely chopped
400 g can diced tomatoes
400 g can gluten-free lentils, drained
small bunch basil leaves, washed and torn
freshly ground black pepper
1 cup (100 g) grated Parmesan cheese
1 cup low GI gluten-free wholemeal breadcrumbs

To serve
wilted baby spinach

1. Preheat the oven to 180°C.

2. Grease an oven tray with a little of the olive oil. Brush some olive oil over the base of the mushrooms and place them on the tray.

3. Heat the remaining oil in a large non-stick frying pan over medium heat. Add the mushroom stems, onion, garlic and capsicum. Reduce the heat and cook, stirring occasionally, for 10 minutes or until the onions are soft and golden. Stir in the diced tomatoes, then add the lentils and basil and stir gently until the mixture is well combined and heated through. Season with pepper and set aside.

4. Process the Parmesan cheese and breadcrumbs to fine crumbs. Spoon the lentil mixture into the mushroom 'cups' and top each one with the breadcrumb mixture.

5. Place tray in the oven and bake for 15 minutes or until the topping is crisp and golden and the mushrooms are cooked through. (Cooking time will vary a little depending on the size of the mushrooms.)

6. Place a little wilted spinach on each plate, top with a mushroom and serve.

PER SERVE

1171 kJ; 14 g fat (including 4 g saturated fat); 6 g fibre; 14 g protein; 23 g carbohydrate

Chapter 8: Snacks and treats

Snacks prevent us from becoming too hungry and reduce the likelihood of overeating when meal times come around. The key is to keep them healthy and quick and easy to prepare.

Apple and Pecan Muffins

Low GI baking is a challenge, surpassed only by low GI gluten-free baking! Diane Temple, our recipe tester, will testify to this. Here we boost the fibre and lower the GI with ingredients such as psyllium husks, banana, apple and brown rice flour. Sifting is the secret of successful gluten-free baking. These muffins remain fresh for a day. Freezing will keep them for a longer time.

Makes 12 **Preparation time** 25 minutes
Cooking time 20 minutes + cooling time

canola oil spray
¾ cup (110 g) rice flour
½ cup (70 g) brown rice flour
½ cup (70 g) gluten-free cornflour
¼ cup (25 g) soy flour
2 teaspoons gluten-free baking powder
1 teaspoon bicarbonate of soda
1 teaspoon xanthan gum
1 tablespoon psyllium husks
½ cup (110 g) caster sugar
1 egg
1 tablespoon canola oil
1 teaspoon vanilla essence
½ cup (125 ml) reduced-fat milk
1 small banana, mashed (about ⅓ cup)
1 large green apple, peeled, cored and diced (about 1 cup)
⅓ cup (40 g) roughly chopped pecans

1 Preheat the oven to 180°C. Spray a 12-hole (each ⅓ cup capacity) muffin pan with canola oil spray.

2 In a large mixing bowl, sift together the rice flour, brown rice flour, cornflour, soy flour, baking powder, bicarbonate of soda and xanthan gum. Stir to mix well then sift a second time into another large bowl. Stir in the psyllium husks and sugar.

3 In a smaller bowl, whisk together the egg, oil, vanilla essence, milk and banana. Pour this mixture into the dry ingredients, add the apple and pecans, and stir well to combine.

4 Spoon the mixture evenly into the muffin holes and smooth over the top of each hole with a palette knife. Bake for 18–20 minutes or until light golden and a skewer inserted into the centre comes out clean. Leave in pan for 5 minutes before turning out onto a wire rack to cool.

PER MUFFIN
742 kJ; 5 g fat (including 0.5 g saturated fat); 2 g fibre; 4 g protein; 30 g carbohydrate

Cherry Chocolate Muffins

These muffins remain fresh for a day. Freezing will keep them for a longer time.

Makes 12 **Preparation time** 20 minutes
Cooking time 15 minutes + cooling time

canola oil spray
⅔ cup (90 g) brown rice flour
½ cup (70 g) gluten-free cornflour
1½ teaspoons gluten-free baking powder
½ teaspoon bicarbonate of soda
1 teaspoon xanthan gum
1 tablespoon psyllium husks
⅓ cup (75 g) caster sugar
⅓ cup (45 g) rice bran cereal
⅔ cup (110 g) dried cherries
⅓ cup (25 g) shredded coconut
¼ cup (45 g) milk choc bits
1 egg, lightly beaten
½ cup (125 ml) low fat milk
2 tablespoons canola oil
1 teaspoon vanilla essence

1 Preheat the oven to 180°C. Spray a 12-hole (each ⅓ cup capacity) muffin pan with canola oil spray.

2 In a large mixing bowl, sift together the brown rice flour, cornflour, baking powder, bicarbonate of soda and xanthan gum and stir to mix well. Sift a second time into another large bowl. Stir in the psyllium husks, sugar, rice bran cereal, cherries, coconut and choc bits.

3 In smaller bowl, whisk together the egg, milk, oil and vanilla. Add the egg mixture to the dry ingredients and stir well to combine.

4 Spoon the mixture evenly into the muffin holes and smooth the top of each with a palette knife. Bake for 15 minutes or until golden and a skewer inserted into the centre comes out clean. Leave in pan for 5 minutes before turning out onto a wire rack to cool.

VARIATIONS

Omit the cherries and try:
- ⅔ cup fruit medley with the coconut and ¼ cup white choc bits instead of the milk choc bits
- ⅔ cup chopped dried apricots with the coconut and ¼ cup dark choc bits (omit milk choc bits), or
- ⅔ cup chopped figs, ⅔ cup toasted flaked almonds (omit coconut) and ¼ cup dark choc bits (omit milk choc bits).

PER MUFFIN

790 kJ; 7 g fat (including 2.5 g saturated fat); 2 g fibre; 3 g protein; 30 g carbohydrate

Corn, Carrot and Onion Muffins

These muffins are quick to prepare and are a delicious snack. Enjoy them as a light lunch with a side serving of salad. They remain fresh for a day. Freezing will keep them for a longer time.

Makes 15 **Preparation time** 25 minutes
Cooking time 25 minutes + cooling time

canola oil spray
⅔ cup (110 g) rice flour
⅓ cup (45 g) gluten-free cornflour
⅓ cup (35 g) soy flour
2 teaspoons gluten-free baking powder
1 teaspoon bicarbonate of soda
1 teaspoon xanthan gum
2 teaspoons rice bran
2 teaspoons psyllium husks
1 cup (170 g) polenta
2½ tablespoons caster sugar
310 g can corn kernels, drained
3 spring onions, sliced
½ cup coarsely grated carrot (about 1 small carrot)
2 tablespoons chopped parsley
¼ cup (60 ml) canola oil
1½ cups (375 ml) buttermilk
1 egg

1. Preheat the oven to 190°C. You will need two 12-hole (each ⅓ cup capacity) muffin pans. Spray 15 of the holes with canola oil spray.

2. In a large mixing bowl, sift together the rice flour, cornflour, soy flour, baking powder, bicarbonate of soda, xanthan gum and rice bran. Stir to combine then sift a second time into another large bowl. Mix in psyllium, polenta and sugar. Add the vegetables and parsley, and stir well to combine.

3. In a smaller bowl, whisk together the oil, buttermilk and egg. Pour into the dry ingredients and vegetables, and stir until just combined.

4. Spoon the mixture evenly into 15 muffin holes, smoothing the top of each with a palette knife. Bake for 20–25 minutes or until tops are slightly golden and a skewer inserted into the centre comes out clean. Leave in pan for 5 minutes before turning out onto a wire rack to cool.

VARIATION
- You can substitute 1 cup fresh or frozen corn kernels for the canned corn.

PER MUFFIN
680 kJ; 5 g fat (including 1 g saturated fat); 1 g fibre; 5 g protein; 24 g carbohydrate

Banana Walnut Loaf

Fruit breads such as this make a satisfying after-school snack and are handy to toast for breakfast. Slice and serve warm or toasted topped with margarine or ricotta cheese. Light cream cheese or ricotta mixed with a little orange zest makes a delicious topping for this loaf.

Makes 12 slices **Preparation time** 25 minutes
Cooking time 40 minutes + cooling time

1 cup (150 g) rice flour
½ cup (70 g) gluten-free cornflour
½ cup (55 g) soy flour
2 teaspoons gluten-free baking powder
1 teaspoon bicarbonate of soda
1 teaspoon xanthan gum
1½ teaspoons cinnamon
2 teaspoons psyllium husks
2 eggs
⅓ cup (75 g) caster sugar
¼ cup (60 ml) canola oil
¼ cup (60 ml) unsweetened cloudy apple juice
1 teaspoon vanilla essence
1 cup mashed banana (about 2–3 bananas, depending on size)
1 cup (120 g) coarsely chopped walnuts

1 Preheat the oven to 180°C. Grease and line a 24 cm × 12 cm-base loaf pan.

2 In a large mixing bowl, sift together the rice flour, cornflour, soy flour, baking powder, bicarbonate of soda, xanthan gum and cinnamon into a large bowl. Stir to combine and then sift a second time into another large bowl. Stir in psyllium husks and make a well in the centre.

3 In a smaller bowl, whisk together the eggs, sugar, oil, apple juice and vanilla. Add the mashed banana and whisk again to combine well. Pour into the well in the dry ingredients and stir, using a wooden spoon, until combined. Stir in the walnuts.

4 Pour the mixture into the prepared pan, levelling the top with a palette knife. Bake for 40 minutes or until cooked and a skewer inserted into the centre comes out clean. Leave in pan for 5 minutes before turning the loaf out onto a wire rack to cool.

PER SLICE
1060 kJ; 14 g fat (including 1 g saturated fat); 1.5 g fibre; 7 g protein; 28 g carbohydrate

Fruit Loaf

We are often asked what can be done to lower the GI of baked foods. This recipe is a good example – it replaces some of the flour with plenty of our favourite low GI ingredients, including cloudy apple juice, dried fruit and rice bran cereal. Cover cake with foil if the top of the cake darkens during baking.

Makes 12 slices **Preparation time** 25 minutes
Cooking time 35 minutes + cooling time

½ cup (125 ml) unsweetened cloudy apple juice
¾ cup (130 g) sultanas
1 cup (140 g) diced dried apricots
1 cup (120 g) rice flour
⅓ cup (45 g) gluten-free cornflour
⅓ cup (40 g) besan (chickpea) flour
2 teaspoons gluten-free baking powder
1 teaspoon bicarbonate of soda
1 teaspoon xanthan gum
3 teaspoons mixed spice
1 tablespoon psyllium husks
½ cup (100 g) firmly packed brown sugar
½ cup (60 g) rice bran cereal, lightly crushed
2 eggs, lightly beaten
2 tablespoons canola oil
½ cup (125 ml) reduced-fat milk
⅓ cup (70 g) diced pitted prunes

1 Preheat the oven to 180°C. Grease and line the base of a 24 cm × 12 cm-base loaf pan.

2 Heat the apple juice in a small saucepan and bring just to the boil. Add the sultanas and apricots, remove from heat, stir and set aside.

3 In a large mixing bowl, sift together the rice flour, cornflour, besan flour, baking powder, bicarbonate of soda, xanthan gum and mixed spice. Stir to combine and then sift a second time into another large bowl. Stir in the psyllium husks, sugar and crushed bran cereal and mix well to combine. Make a well in the centre.

4 In a smaller bowl, whisk together the eggs, oil and milk. Pour into the well the dry ingredients, then add the dried fruit and apple juice mixture, and the prunes. Stir with a wooden spoon until well combined.

5 Pour the mixture into the prepared loaf pan and smooth the top with a palette knife. Bake for 25–30 minutes or until golden and a skewer inserted into the centre comes out clean. Leave in pan for 5 minutes before turning out onto a wire rack to cool.

PER SLICE
886 kJ; 5 g fat (including 0.5 g saturated fat); 2.8 g fibre; 4 g protein; 38 g carbohydrate

Low GI, gluten-free baking tips

- Sift the gluten-free flours twice as we suggest – it gives the dry ingredients a good airing.
- When baking, sift the dry ingredients first, and then most of the work is done!
- The ingredient list may seem long, but we use a mixture of gluten-free flours plus ingredients such as baking powder and xanthan gum to help with texture, as well as rice bran and psyllium husks to increase the fibre content.

Brownies

There's nothing like a batch of brownies at the end of a long day. They make a wonderful after-school treat or a delicious dessert to nibble on with coffee or tea. As we say at the beginning of this chapter, treats are important – as long as they're just that, not an everyday food. As a finishing touch, place 2 teaspoons of gluten-free icing sugar into a small, fine strainer and shake gently over each one.

Makes 12 slices **Preparation time** 20 minutes
Cooking time 25 minutes + cooling time

⅓ cup (45 g) brown rice flour
⅓ cup (55 g) potato flour
½ teaspoon gluten-free baking powder
¼ teaspoon bicarbonate of soda
¼ teaspoon xanthan gum
¼ cup (30 g) cocoa
⅔ cup (80 g) almond meal
2 teaspoons psyllium husks
100 g dark chocolate (63% cocoa), roughly chopped
100 g reduced-fat margarine
⅓ cup (65 g) brown sugar
1 teaspoon vanilla extract
1 egg
½ cup (125 ml) buttermilk
pure icing sugar or gluten-free icing sugar mixture (optional), to serve

1 Preheat the oven to 180°C. Grease and line a 19 cm × 19 cm-base cake pan.

2 In a large mixing bowl, sift the brown rice flour, potato flour, baking powder, bicarbonate of soda, xanthan gum and cocoa. Stir to combine dry ingredients and sift a second time into another large bowl. Stir in the almond meal and psyllium husks, and set aside.

3 Melt the chocolate, margarine and sugar in a medium–large saucepan on a low heat, stirring until smooth. Remove from the heat and add the vanilla. Stir in the egg and then the dry ingredients mix. Pour in the buttermilk and combine well.

4 Spoon the brownie mixture into the prepared pan, smoothing the top evenly with a palette knife. Bake for 20 minutes or until the top is firm and a skewer inserted into the centre comes out clean. Leave in the pan to cool before dusting with icing sugar, if you wish.

PER BROWNIE WITHOUT ICING SUGAR
795 kJ; 11 g fat (including 4 g saturated fat); 1.5 g fibre; 3 g protein; 18 g carbohydrate

Muesli Nut Biscuits

Crunchy biscuits are very popular in lunchboxes. These ones are packed with nutrients and fibre and, as an after-school snack, will provide an energy boost before kids' sports training or homework. They will keep for a few days in an airtight container. If they become soft, you can 'crisp' them up in a preheated 180°C oven for 4–5 minutes.

Makes about 26 **Preparation time** 20 minutes
Cooking time 25 minutes + cooling time

80 g reduced-fat margarine
¼ cup (60 ml) honey
⅓ cup (45 g) brown rice flour
⅓ cup (45 g) gluten-free cornflour
½ teaspoon gluten-free baking powder
½ teaspoon xanthan gum
1 teaspoon cinnamon
2 tablespoons brown sugar
2 cups gluten-free low GI muesli
2 tablespoons almond meal
¼ cup (35 g) chopped macadamia nuts
¼ cup (30 g) chopped walnuts
1 egg, lightly beaten
½ teaspoon vanilla essence

1. Preheat the oven to 160°C. Line 2 baking trays with baking paper.

2. Melt the margarine and honey in a small saucepan, stirring occasionally. Set aside to cool.

3. In a mixing bowl, sift the brown rice flour, cornflour, baking powder, xanthan gum and cinnamon. Stir to combine, then sift a second time into another bowl. Stir through the sugar, muesli, almond meal, macadamia nuts and walnuts.

4. Pour the cooled margarine mix into the muesli mix, add the egg and the vanilla, and stir with a wooden spoon to combine.

5. Take 1 tablespoon of the mix, shape into a ball, flatten slightly and place on a baking tray. Continue with remaining mix. Bake for 18–20 minutes, swapping trays halfway during cooking, or until golden. Leave on trays for 10 minutes before transferring to a wire rack to cool.

PER BISCUIT
466 kJ; 7 g fat (including 2 g saturated fat); 2 g fibre; 2 g protein; 10 g carbohydrate

No-bake Chocolate Clusters

This is a recipe for making your own fruit chocolates! You will achieve the best results with a good-quality chocolate – one with 63% cocoa solids is ideal. A darker chocolate (around 70%) may be too bitter. You can buy amaranth breakfast cereal in health food stores and the health food aisle of supermarkets.

Makes about 50 **Preparation time** 10 minutes
Cooking time 5 minutes + setting time

400 g dark chocolate (63% cocoa)
½ cup (90 g) sultanas
½ cup (80 g) craisins (dried cranberries)
½ cup (70 g) chopped dried apricots
½ cup (50 g) chopped dried apples
¼ cup (10 g) amaranth breakfast cereal (optional)

1 Melt the chocolate in a medium-sized bowl over a saucepan of simmering water, stirring occasionally, until the chocolate has melted and is smooth.

2 In a small bowl, combine the sultanas, craisins, apricots, apples and amaranth (if using). Add to the melted chocolate and stir to combine and coat the fruit.

3 Place a heaped teaspoonful of the mix on a lined baking tray. Repeat with the remaining mixture, placing the clusters 3–4 cm apart. Place in the refrigerator to set. Store the clusters in an airtight container in the refrigerator.

PER CLUSTER WITHOUT AMARANTH
220 kJ; 2.5 g fat (including 2 g saturated fat); 0.5 g fibre; 0.5 g protein; 7 g carbohydrate

Apricot Nut Slice

Diane originally created this for our free online newsletter, GI News, and it was so popular with our readers there, we decided to include it in this book. The GI is probably moderate as it uses sweet gluten-free biscuits in the base.

Makes 12 pieces **Preparation time** 10 minutes **Cooking time** 25 minutes

120 g plain, sweet gluten-free biscuits, crushed into crumbs
⅓ cup (60 g) brown rice flour
⅓ cup (35 g) hazelnut meal
1 egg white
40 g reduced-fat margarine, melted

Filling

200 g dried apricots
60 g dried cherries
1 cup (250 ml) water
2 teaspoons caster sugar
30 g flaked almonds

1. Pre-heat the oven to 180°C. Grease a 26 cm × 16 cm-base slice pan. Line the base and the 2 long sides with baking paper and extend the paper a few centimetres above the edge of the pan to help with removing the slice when it is cooked and cooled.

2. To make the base: combine the biscuit crumbs, flour and hazelnut meal in a medium bowl. Whisk the egg white until slightly foamy. Add the margarine and egg white to the crumbs and mix together using your fingers to combine. Press the mixture into the base of the prepared pan. Bake for 10 minutes or until base is lightly browned.

3. For the topping: place the apricots, cherries and water in a small saucepan and bring to the boil. Simmer for 10 minutes until the fruit is soft, stirring occasionally to break up the fruit. Mix through the sugar. Spread the filling evenly over the cooked base. Sprinkle the flaked almonds over the top.

4. Bake the slice for 15 minutes or until the almonds are lightly toasted. Leave in the pan to cool. Slice when cold and store in an airtight container.

PER PIECE
741 kJ; 8 g fat (including 1.5 g saturated fat); 2.5 g fibre; 3 g protein; 23 g carbohydrate

Take 5

5 quick snacks

- Fresh fruit salad
- A handful of fresh or frozen grapes
- Celery, cucumber or carrot sticks, or capsicum wedges with hommous or a yoghurt-based dip
- Smoothie (see our recipes, pages 99–101)
- Hommous on a gluten-free cracker

5 grab 'n' run snacks

- A piece of fruit, such as a juicy orange, a small banana, a large peach or pear
- A handful of dried fruit and nut mix
- A handful of dried apricots or apple rings, sultanas or raisins
- A tub of low fat yoghurt or a dairy dessert
- A small piece of low fat cheese or a cheese stick

5 warming snacks

- A piece of corn on the cob
- A mug of gluten-free vegetable soup with a slice of gluten-free toast
- A toasted sandwich made with low GI gluten-free bread
- A small can of baked beans or creamed corn
- A small serving of gluten-free noodles with vegetables

5 thirst-quenching snacks

- A small glass (200 ml) of fruit juice
- A glass of low fat milk or calcium-enriched gluten-free soy milk
- A glass of iced water with a twist of lemon or lime
- A smoothie (see our recipes, pages 99–101)
- A café latte with low fat milk

Chapter 9

Light meals and lunches

Refuelling at lunchtime helps you maintain your energy levels and concentration through the afternoon. It also reduces the temptation to snack mindlessly on an entire packet of chips later in the day.

Beef and Bean Fajitas

This can be one of those 'assemble your own' meals. Arrange the ingredients attractively on a big platter or in several small bowls and go for it.

Makes 12 **Preparation time** 25 minutes **Cooking time** 15 minutes

1 tablespoon olive oil
250 g lean rump steak, thinly sliced
1 red (Spanish) onion, sliced
1 red capsicum, sliced
1 yellow capsicum, sliced
1–2 jalapeno chillies (optional), seeded and finely chopped
¼ teaspoon chilli powder
2 teaspoons sweet paprika
1 teaspoon ground cumin
1 teaspoon ground coriander
juice of 1 lime
2 tablespoons tomato paste
½ teaspoon sugar
¼ cup chopped coriander leaves
400 g can kidney beans, rinsed and drained
125 g can corn kernels, drained

To serve
12 gluten-free white corn tortillas
1 quantity Easy Guacamole (see Basics)
½ cup (50 g) grated low fat tasty cheese
mixed salad leaves

1. Heat 2 teaspoons oil in a large frying pan. Add the meat and stir-fry for 3–4 minutes or until brown. Remove from the pan and set aside.

2. Add the remaining oil to the pan, add the onion, capsicums and chillies, if using, and cook for 3 minutes. Stir in the chilli powder, paprika, cumin, coriander, lime juice, tomato paste and sugar. Return all the meat to the pan and cook for 2–3 minutes. Stir in the coriander leaves, kidney beans and corn kernels, and stir until heated through.

3. Heat the tortillas following the packet instructions (either in the microwave for 30 seconds or wrap in foil and warm in the oven for a few minutes).

4. On each tortilla, place some of the beef mixture on one side, add 1 tablespoon guacamole, a little cheese and salad leaves, and roll up. Alternatively, arrange the tortillas on a large platter, and in several bowls the beef mixture, guacamole, salad leaves and cheese, and let everyone make their own.

PER FAJITA WITH GUACAMOLE
900 kJ; 10 g fat (including 3 g saturated fat); 3.5 g fibre; 10 g protein; 20 g carbohydrate

Chicken Nuggets with Salad

These tangy nuggets are great for lunch or a light meal. They are also perfect for parties or finger-food events. Diane's daughter, Ava, thinks that they are so delicious they should be served with a big sign reading 'For Kids Only'.

Makes 16 **Preparation time** 15 minutes **Cooking time** 10 minutes

½ cup dried gluten-free breadcrumbs
1½ tablespoons sesame seeds
400 g chicken breast, chopped roughly
3 teaspoons reduced-salt gluten-free tamari
3 teaspoons gluten-free plum sauce

To serve
vegetable sticks
cherry tomatoes
gluten-free tomato sauce or gluten-free sweet chilli sauce

1. Preheat the oven to 180°C. Line a baking tray with baking paper.

2. Mix the breadcrumbs and sesame seeds together and place on a large flat dish.

3. Place the chicken, tamari and plum sauce in a food processor and process until well mixed and the chicken is minced.

4. Wet your hands and take a tablespoon of the chicken mixture, form into a disc about the size of a matchbox and roll it in the breadcrumb mix. Place the nugget on the baking tray and continue with the remaining mix.

5. Bake nuggets for 10–12 minutes or until chicken is cooked through and the crumbs are golden and crunchy. Serve with sauce for dipping, along with cherry tomatoes and vegetable sticks such as carrot, cucumber, celery and capsicum.

PER NUGGET WITHOUT VEGETABLES
221 kJ; 2.5 g fat (including 0.5 g saturated fat); 0.5 g fibre; 6 g protein; 2 g carbohydrate

Chicken Tacos

Tacos are another 'make your own' favourite. Or you can also assemble them beforehand and serve them ready-made on a large platter. We also include a variation for Chilli Bean Tacos for vegetarians.

Serves 4 **Preparation time** 20 minutes **Cooking time** 20 minutes

2 teaspoons olive oil
2 cloves garlic, crushed
250 g chicken mince
1½ teaspoons ground cumin
1 teaspoon oregano
¼ teaspoon ground chilli (optional)
½ red capsicum, diced
½ green capsicum, diced
400 g can diced tomatoes
1 tablespoon tomato paste
¼ teaspoon sugar
freshly ground black pepper
400 g can kidney beans, drained and rinsed

To serve

12 gluten-free taco shells
1 quantity Easy Guacamole (see Basics)
2 cups shredded iceberg lettuce
1 cup (100 g) reduced-fat grated tasty cheese
2 tomatoes, diced

1. Heat the oil in a large frying pan, add garlic and chicken, and cook for 3–4 minutes, stirring and breaking up chicken. Add the cumin, oregano and chilli, and cook for 1 minute more. Add the capsicums, canned tomatoes, tomato paste, sugar and pepper, stir, bring to the boil and simmer for 10 minutes. Stir in the kidney beans until heated through.

2. Meanwhile, line a tray with baking paper, place the taco shells on the tray, and bake in the oven for 4–5 minutes or until warm (not hot) and crisp.

3. To serve, fill the shells with the chicken mixture. Top with guacamole, lettuce, cheese and diced tomatoes.

VARIATION

- To make Chilli Bean Tacos, replace the chicken with an extra can of kidney beans or 400 g can drained lentils.

PER TACO WITH SERVING SUGGESTIONS
805 kJ; 10 g fat (including 2.5 g saturated fat); 3 g fibre; 10 g protein; 13 g carbohydrate

Falafel Wraps

Made with chickpeas, falafel are a low GI favourite. And because they are equally tasty hot or cold, they are ideal for lunchboxes and after-school snacks on their own or in a wrap.

Serves 4 (makes 12) **Preparation time** 15 minutes **Cooking time** 20 minutes

400 g can chickpeas, drained and rinsed
2 cloves garlic, chopped
1 teaspoon ground cumin
½ teaspoon ground coriander
2 tablespoons finely chopped parsley
1 tablespoon chopped coriander leaves
½ teaspoon gluten-free baking powder
olive oil spray

To serve

Hommous (see Basics)
4 large gluten-free wraps
Pistachio and Quinoa Tabbouli (see page 147)

1. Preheat the oven to 200°C. Line a baking tray with baking paper.

2. Place the chickpeas and garlic in a food processor and process until fairly smooth. Transfer to a bowl and combine well with the cumin, coriander, chopped parsley, chopped coriander leaves and baking powder.

3. To make the falafel patties, take 1 tablespoon of the mixture, roll into a ball and flatten slightly. Place on the prepared tray. Continue with remaining mixture. Spray the falafel patties with olive oil spray. Bake for 20 minutes, turning the patties over halfway during cooking time. The patties should be slightly crisp on the outside and lightly golden. Transfer to a plate and set aside.

4. Spread 2 tablespoons of hommous over 1 side of each wrap. Top each with about ⅓ cup tabbouli and 3 falafels. Roll up the wraps and serve.

VARIATIONS
- For extra oomph, add a tablespoon of a tangy gluten-free salsa or sauce.
- Serve with tahini rather than hommous.

PER FALAFEL PATTIE
123 kJ; 1 g fat (including 0 g saturated fat); 1 g fibre; 1 g protein; 3 g carbohydrate

Corn and Coriander Fritters

Our timing for this recipe is based on cooking the fritters one at a time. But if you have a very large frying pan, you could cook two at a time.

Serves 4 (makes 8) **Preparation time** 25 minutes **Cooking time** 20 minutes

1 large corn cob (to make 1 cup corn kernels)
½ red capsicum, diced
¼ cup chopped coriander
1 red chilli, de-seeded and finely diced
3 spring onions, thinly sliced
½ cup (80 g) buckwheat flour
1 teaspoon gluten-free baking powder
½ teaspoon paprika
3 eggs, lightly beaten
150 ml buttermilk
freshly ground black pepper
about 2 tablespoons canola oil

To serve

125 g low fat plain yoghurt
1 tablespoon gluten-free sweet chilli sauce
1 tablespoon chopped coriander
green salad with vinaigrette dressing

1 Cut the corn kernels off the cob. Combine the corn, capsicum, coriander, chilli and spring onions in a large bowl, and set aside.

2 Sift the buckwheat flour, baking powder and paprika into a medium bowl, and make a well in the centre.

3 Whisk together the eggs and buttermilk in a smaller bowl, season with freshly ground black pepper and pour into the well the dry ingredient mix. Whisk to combine well. Stir the combined mixture into the vegetables and mix well.

4 Heat 2 teaspoons oil in a non-stick frying pan. Pour in ¼ cup (60 ml) of the mixture and, using a palette knife, spread to around 12 cm in diameter. Cook on a low–medium heat for 1 minute on each side or until light golden-brown. Remove and drain on paper towel. Repeat with the remaining batter, adding 1–2 extra teaspoons of oil as needed to the pan.

5 Meanwhile, mix the yoghurt with the sweet chilli sauce.

6 Place 2 fritters on each plate and serve topped with some yoghurt mix, a sprinkle of chopped coriander and a serving of salad.

VARIATION

- You can substitute a 310 g can of drained corn or 1 cup frozen corn kernels for the corn cob.

PER SERVE WITHOUT SALAD

1291 kJ; 15 g fat (including 2.5 g saturated fat); 2 g fibre; 13 g protein; 15 g carbohydrate

Individual Spanish Tortillas

These little tortillas are a meal in themselves. Canola oil spray works really well, preventing the tortillas from sticking or leaving a mess. Steam the potato and sweet potato rather than boiling, if you prefer.

Makes 8 **Preparation time** 20 minutes
Cooking time 30 minutes + cooling time

canola oil spray
150 g Carisma, Nicola or small chat potatoes, peeled and chopped into 1 cm chunks
200 g orange sweet potato, peeled and chopped into 1 cm chunks
2 teaspoons canola oil
1 small red capsicum, diced
3 rashers (60 g) lean shortcut bacon, all visible fat removed, diced
80 g spinach leaves
6 eggs
½ cup (125 ml) low fat milk
freshly ground black pepper

1. Preheat the oven to 180°C. Spray 8 holes of a 12-hole muffin pan (each ¾ cup capacity) with canola oil spray.

2. Place the potato and sweet potato in a small saucepan of boiling water, and cook for about 8 minutes or until just tender. Drain.

3. In a large frying pan, heat the oil, add the capsicum and bacon, and cook for 1 minute. Add the potato and sweet potato, and brown a little, about 2–3 minutes.

4. Remove from the heat, stir in the spinach, then pour the mixture into a large bowl.

5. Whisk the eggs and milk together in a small bowl, and season. Pour into a jug.

6. Spoon about 2–3 tablespoons of the vegetable mixture into each muffin pan hole. Pour over the egg mixture. Bake for 20 minutes or until just set. Leave in the pan for 5 minutes before turning out onto a wire rack to cool.

VARIATIONS
- Replace the orange sweet potato with butternut pumpkin.
- To make a vegetarian version, omit the bacon. Cook 1 chopped onion for 3–4 minutes, and then add other vegetables.

PER TORTILLA
473 kJ; 5 g fat (including 1.5 g saturated fat); 1 g fibre; 8 g protein; 8 g carbohydrate

Italian Meatballs in Tomato Sauce

This classic family favourite is delicious served with rice and a big crispy green salad. The mince mixture also makes 8 meat patties (using ¼ cup of mixture for each). Grill, pan-fry or barbecue to make the burgers. We used Herbie's Italian Herbs mix for this but give the recipe in Basics a go if you want to make your own.

Serves 4 **Preparation time** 10 minutes **Cooking time** 20 minutes

500 g lean beef mince
⅓ cup fresh gluten-free low GI breadcrumbs
¼ teaspoon chilli powder
1 teaspoon Italian herbs or 1 teaspoon oregano
2 cloves garlic, crushed
¼ cup (60 ml) tomato paste

Tomato sauce

2 cups (500 ml) tomato passata or bottled tomato sauce
1 cup (250 ml) gluten-free reduced-salt chicken stock
1 teaspoon sugar
freshly ground black pepper
2 tablespoons chopped parsley

To serve

1 cup (200 g) low GI rice (e.g. basmati or Doongara Clever rice), cooked
green salad with vinaigrette dressing

1 In a large bowl, combine the mince, breadcrumbs, chilli powder, Italian herb mix, garlic and tomato paste, and mix well. Roll heaped tablespoons of the mixture into balls. Chill.

2 Meanwhile, place the passata, stock, sugar and some pepper into a medium saucepan and bring to the boil. Arrange the meatballs in the sauce, reduce the heat and simmer, uncovered, for 15 minutes or until meatballs are cooked through. Stir in the parsley.

3 Serve with rice and salad.

PER SERVING WITH MEATBALLS, SAUCE AND RICE
1315 kJ; 11 g fat (including 5 g saturated fat); 2 g fibre; 29 g protein; 25 g carbohydrate

Salmon and Pumpkin Patties with Butter Bean Salad

To make the amount of mashed pumpkin you need for this recipe, boil, steam or microwave 100 grams peeled butternut pumpkin. Drain off any excess liquid and mash with a fork.

Makes 4 patties **Preparation time** 25 minutes **Chilling time** 30 minutes **Cooking time** 25 minutes

200 g can pink salmon, drained
400 g can butter beans, drained
⅓ cup mashed butternut pumpkin
2 spring onions, chopped
2 teaspoons rice bran
½ teaspoon gluten-free curry powder
1 tablespoon brown rice flour
2 teaspoons canola oil
80 g wild rocket

Butter Bean Salad
2 tablespoons balsamic vinegar
1 tablespoon extra virgin olive oil
1 small red capsicum, chopped
½ small red onion, diced
1 small avocado, diced

1. In a medium bowl, mash the salmon and ½ cup butter beans with a fork. (Reserve the remaining beans for the salad.)

2. Mix in the pumpkin, spring onions, bran and curry powder. Divide the mix into 4 portions and shape each into a pattie about 8–9 cm across. Chill in the refrigerator for 30 minutes.

3. Meanwhile, preheat the oven to 180°C. Line a baking tray with baking paper. Dust the patties with brown rice flour. In a large frying pan, heat the canola oil, add the patties and cook on a medium heat for 1 minute each side or until just golden brown. Place the patties on the baking tray and cook in the oven for 20–25 minutes or until firm.

4 To make the Butter Bean Salad, whisk together the balsamic vinegar and oil. Combine the capsicum, onion, avocado and reserved butter beans in a small bowl. Toss with half of the balsamic dressing.

5 Place the rocket in a bowl and toss with the remaining dressing. Divide the rocket equally among four serving plates, top each with a salmon pattie and a large spoonful of butter bean salad.

PER SERVE
1311 kJ; 24 g fat (including 5 g saturated fat); 3.5 g fibre; 15 g protein; 7 g carbohydrate

Chicken Mango Rice Paper Rolls

Makes 12 **Preparation time** 30 minutes **Cooking time** 10 minutes

1 x 250 g skinless chicken breast
50 g bean thread noodles
1 mango, peeled and cut into short strips
50 g (about 6) snow peas, trimmed and sliced diagonally in half
¼ cup shredded mint
12 round 22 cm rice papers

Dipping Sauce
⅓ cup (80 ml) lime juice
1 tablespoon fish sauce
1 tablespoon caster sugar

1 Put about 1½ cups (375 ml) water in a small saucepan (enough to cover the chicken) and bring to the boil. Add the chicken, reduce the heat, and simmer, covered, for 10 minutes. Set aside to cool in the pan. When cool enough to handle, shred and then refrigerate.

2 Place the noodles in a heatproof bowl and cover with boiling water. Leave for 3–4 minutes or until soft, then drain. Rinse the noodles under running water to cool, drain again and cut into short lengths (1–2 cm).

3 To make the Dipping Sauce, combine all ingredients in a bowl and stir until sugar dissolves. Set aside.

4 Place all filling ingredients on a bench. Dip the wrappers one at a time in a shallow bowl of warm water for 10–15 seconds or until just soft. Drain off excess water and place on a clean surface.

5 Place about 1 tablespoon shredded chicken, 1 heaped teaspoon noodles, 2 strips of mango, 2 pieces of snow pea and 1 teaspoon mint on the rice paper, about 3 cm in from the base. Fold up the bottom of the wrapper, then fold in the sides and roll up to enclose the filling. Place on a tray and cover with paper towels. Continue with remaining filling and wrappers. Serve the rolls on a platter with the Dipping Sauce.

PER ROLL WITH DIPPING SAUCE
314 kJ; 1 g fat (including 0.5 g saturated fat); 0.5 g fibre; 6 g protein; 10 g carbohydrate

Carrot, Avocado and Snow Pea Rice Paper Rolls

Squeeze some lime juice over the avocado after it has been sliced to prevent it from turning brown.

Makes 12 **Preparation time** 30 minutes

50 g bean thread noodles
1 small carrot, cut into short, thin sticks
1 avocado, sliced into short, thin slices
squeeze of lime juice for the avocado
½ bunch garlic chives, cut into 3
50 g (about 6) snow peas, sliced diagonally in half
50 g snow pea sprouts, ends trimmed
12 round 22 cm rice papers

Dipping Sauce
3 tablespoons gluten-free sweet chilli sauce
3 tablespoons lime juice
2 teaspoons reduced-salt gluten-free tamari

1. Place bean thread noodles in a heatproof bowl and cover with boiling water. Leave for 3–4 minutes or until noodles are soft, then drain. Rinse under running water to cool, then drain and cut noodles into short lengths (1–2 cm).

2. To make the Dipping Sauce, combine all ingredients in a bowl and set aside.

3. Place all the filling ingredients on a bench. Half-fill a large bowl with warm water. Dip one wrapper in the water for 10–15 seconds or until it is just soft. Drain off excess water and place on a clean surface.

4. Place a heaped teaspoon of noodles, and a few pieces of each of the carrot, avocado, garlic chives, snow peas and sprouts on the wrapper, about 3 cm in from the base. Fold up the bottom of the wrapper, then fold in the sides and roll up to enclose filling. Place on a tray and cover with paper towels. Continue with remaining filling and wrappers.

5. Serve the rolls on a platter with the dipping sauce.

PER ROLL WITH DIPPING SAUCE
360 kJ; 5 g fat (including 1 g saturated fat); 1 g fibre; 2 g protein; 8 g carbohydrate

Tangy Tuna Rice Paper Rolls

Makes 12 **Preparation time** 30 minutes

50 g bean thread noodles
185 g can tuna in brine or spring water, drained
½ cup grated carrot (about 1 small carrot)
½ cup shredded Chinese cabbage
2 spring onions, thinly sliced
1 tablespoon chopped mint
¼ cup (60 ml) lemon juice
2 teaspoons sesame oil
3 teaspoons honey
12 round 22 cm rice papers

Dipping Sauce
⅓ cup (80 ml) tomato sauce
3 teaspoons reduced-salt gluten-free tamari

1. Place bean thread noodles in a heatproof bowl and cover with boiling water. Leave for 3–4 minutes or until noodles are soft, then drain. Rinse under running water to cool, drain and then cut noodles into small lengths (1–2 cm).

2. In a large bowl, combine tuna, carrot, cabbage, spring onions and mint, and mix well.

3. In a small bowl, whisk together the juice, oil and honey. Pour over the tuna mix and stir through.

4. To make the Dipping Sauce, combine the ingredients in a bowl. Set aside.

5. Half fill a large bowl with warm water. Dip one wrapper in the water for 10–15 seconds or until just soft. Drain off excess water and place on a clean surface.

6. Place ¼ cup of the tuna mixture on the wrapper, about 3 cm in from the base. Fold up the bottom of the wrapper, then fold in the sides and roll up to enclose the filling. Place on a tray and cover with paper towels. Continue with remaining filling and wrappers.

7. Serve the rolls on a platter with the Dipping Sauce.

PER ROLL WITH DIPPING SAUCE
292 kJ; 1 g fat (including 0.5 g saturated fat); 0.5 g fibre; 5 g protein; 9 g carbohydrate

Lunchbox tips

Although gluten-free breads are improving in texture, there's a general consensus that they aren't ideal for sandwiches, unless toasted. So when packing lunch, try these ideas:

- Mini vegetable frittatas (include vegetables such as corn, sweet potato, a few chickpeas, green peas, zucchini and capsicum)
- Vegetable muffins
- Tuna or salmon and rice slice (mix together low GI rice, tuna or salmon, peas, sweetcorn and egg, top with grated cheese, bake in oven, and cut into squares)
- Pumpkin and salmon patties
- Homemade pasta salad with gluten-free pasta and plenty of vegies
- Homemade potato salad with small chat or Nicola potatoes, corn kernels, peas and capsicum strips
- Lentil and vegetable soup, or chicken and corn soup
- Baked beans with corn thins
- Vietnamese rice paper rolls
- California or sushi rolls
- Corn tortilla wrap spread with avocado and filled with Mexican beans, shredded lettuce, diced cucumber and grated cheese
- Gluten-free wrap filled with falafel, hommous, and Pistachio and Quinoa Tabbouli, and
- For a quick rice salad, use ready-cooked brown or basmati rice tossed in a vinaigrette dressing with corn kernels, red capsicum strips and spring onions.

Add to any of these meals a piece of fruit or two, and a snack for morning-tea break, and the lunchbox is ready to go.

Sushi with Three Fillings

SunRice Doongara CleverRice™ is nearly as good as using sushi rice except it won't be quite as sticky. The main difference is that it doesn't need to be washed. To make a dipping sauce to serve, mix a little reduced-salt tamari and wasabi together, to taste. The marinade from the tofu is also nice as a dipping sauce.

Preparation time 15 minutes
Cooking time 20 minutes + 10 minutes standing time

1 cup (210 g) SunRice Doongara CleverRice™
¼ cup (60 ml) rice wine vinegar
1 tablespoon caster sugar
8 sheets toasted nori

Avocado and Tofu Filling
Makes 4 rolls

100 g firm tofu, cut into 2 slices, then cut again in half lengthways
2 tablespoons reduced-salt gluten-free tamari
2 tablespoons mirin
1 clove garlic, crushed
½ avocado, thinly sliced
1 Lebanese cucumber, cut into short strips

Salmon Filling
Makes 2 rolls

50 g smoked salmon, sliced
½ avocado, thinly sliced

Tuna Filling
Makes 2 rolls

95 g can (or nearest size) tuna in brine or spring water, drained
1 tablespoon gluten-free low fat mayonnaise or plain yoghurt
1 dab of wasabi paste, or to taste
½ Lebanese cucumber, de-seeded, cut into long strips

1 To marinate the tofu for the avocado and tofu filling, place the tofu in a small dish. Combine the tamari, mirin and garlic in a separate small dish, pour over the tofu and place in the refrigerator to marinate for about 30 minutes. The longer you can leave it the better.

2 Place the rice in a medium-sized saucepan with 1½ cups (375 ml) water. Bring to the boil, then reduce the heat, cover and simmer for 15 minutes. Remove from heat and stand for 10 minutes.

3 Gently heat vinegar and sugar, stirring, until sugar dissolves. Gently fold the vinegar mixture into the rice. Spread rice over a tray, cover with plastic wrap and leave to cool.

4 Run a bamboo sushi mat under

water, shake off the excess water and place on a flat surface. Place one nori sheet, rough side up and with a long end closest to you, on the mat. Using wet hands, place a quarter of the rice on the sheet, and pat down to cover the sheet, leaving 4 cm at the top of the sheet. Press the rice firmly down on the sheet and make a slight indent in the rice 4 cm in from the bottom of the sheet closest to you.

5 To make the avocado and tofu-filled rolls, drain the tofu from the marinade. Place two pieces of tofu in the indent, then a few slices of avocado and strips of cucumber. Roll up the sushi. Repeat to make the other rolls.

6 To make the salmon-filled rolls, place half the smoked salmon and half the avocado in the indent along the rice. Using the bamboo mat, firmly roll up the sushi. Remove the mat. Using a wet knife, cut the roll into thick, equal slices. Repeat to make a second roll.

7 To make the tuna-filled rolls, combine the tuna with the mayonnaise and wasabi. Place half the cucumber strips and half the tuna in the indent along the rice and roll up the sushi. Repeat to make the second roll.

PER ROLL (CUT INTO 4 PIECES SUSHI)
Avocado and Tofu: 1279 kJ; 9 g fat (including 2 g saturated fat); 2 g fibre; 8 g protein; 47 g carbohydrate
Salmon: 1279 kJ; 9 g fat (including 2 g saturated fat); 2 g fibre; 8 g protein; 47 g carbohydrate
Tuna: 1194 kJ; 3 g fat (including 1 g saturated fat); 1 g fibre; 15 g protein; 48 g carbohydrate

Chapter 10: Salads and soups

For a relaxing, informal meal in a bowl, you can't beat a soup or salad for healthy satisfaction.

Thai Beef Salad with Chilli Lime Dressing

This is a tangy light meal and the leftovers are ideal for lunch or as a snack. It's an easy recipe to modify to suit your taste. Add some more vegetables if you like, or rice vermicelli for a more substantial salad. Leftover salad can be stored in an airtight container in the refrigerator for up to 1 day.

Serves 4 **Preparation time** 20 minutes
Cooking time 10 minutes + resting time

canola oil spray
4 small (about 100 g each) lean beef steaks
50 g dried rice vermicelli
1 medium carrot, peeled and cut into thin strips
1 medium Lebanese cucumber, cut into thin strips
1 medium red capsicum, cut into thin strips
1 cup (90 g) bean sprouts
1 bunch mint, leaves picked and roughly chopped
1 bunch coriander, leaves picked, roughly chopped

Chilli Lime Dressing

2 tablespoons lime juice
2 tablespoons fish sauce
1 tablespoon grated palm sugar or raw sugar
2 teaspoons white wine vinegar
1 small fresh red chilli, very finely chopped

1. Preheat a chargrill or heavy-based frying pan on medium–high and lightly spray with canola oil. Cook the steaks for 3–4 minutes on each side (depending on thickness) or to your liking.

2. Wrap in foil and set aside for 10 minutes to rest before slicing finely, cutting diagonally across the grain.

3. Meanwhile, prepare the rice vermicelli according to packet instructions. Drain well and cut into short lengths.

4. To make the Chilli Lime Dressing, whisk all ingredients together in a small bowl. It should have a slightly sour taste with just a touch of sweetness and a little heat. If you like it tangier, add extra fish sauce, lime juice or sugar to taste.

5. In a large serving bowl, combine the beef, rice vermicelli, carrot, cucumber, capsicum, bean sprouts, mint and coriander. Toss well with the Chilli Lime Dressing and serve.

VARIATION

- For a vegetarian meal, replace the beef with an equivalent amount of marinated tofu.

PER SERVE

986 kJ; 8 g fat (including 2.5 g saturated fat); 2.5 g fibre; 24 g protein; 16 g carbohydrate

Warm Potato Salad with Herbs and Toasted Hazelnuts

The Dijon Dressing in this recipe is a favourite of our tester, Diane Temple. Using two vinegars does make a difference. Store leftover salad in an airtight container in the refrigerator for up to 1 day.

Serves 4 **Preparation time** 15 minutes **Cooking time** 10–15 minutes

about 500 g Carisma, Nicola or small chat potatoes, scrubbed and cut into thick slices

400 g can red kidney beans, drained and rinsed

1 avocado, peeled and sliced

2 spring onions, finely sliced

2 tablespoons roughly chopped flatleaf (Italian) parsley

2 tablespoons lightly toasted chopped hazelnuts

Dijon Dressing

2 tablespoons olive oil

1 tablespoon white wine vinegar

1 tablespoon cider vinegar

1 teaspoon Dijon mustard

½ teaspoon (or to taste) caster sugar

1 small clove garlic, crushed (optional)

pinch salt (optional)

freshly ground black pepper

1. Steam the potatoes, covered, for 10 minutes or until tender. Drain well.

2. Meanwhile, to make the Dijon Dressing, whisk all ingredients together in a small bowl.

3. Place the warm potato slices in a large serving bowl, add the beans, pour over the dressing and stir through the potatoes so they are well coated with the dressing. Add the avocado slices, onions and parsley, toss gently to combine, top with the toasted hazelnuts, and serve.

VARIATION

- Replace the red kidney beans with lima beans; the avocado with 2 medium beetroot, roasted and diced; and the parsley with dill.

PER SERVE

1625 kJ; 26 g fat (including 4.5 g saturated fat); 8 g fibre; 9 g protein; 26 g carbohydrate

Chicken Pasta Salad with Mango Salsa

Most (but not all) gluten-free pastas are made from corn or rice flour and have a high GI which is why we like to combine them with ingredients we know will help reduce the overall GI.

Serves 4 **Preparation time** 20 minutes **Cooking time** 20 minutes

1 x 250 g skinless chicken breast
1 tablespoon olive oil
1–2 teaspoons Madras Curry Blend (see Basics)
150 g gluten-free pasta shells, or your favourite shape
1 Lebanese cucumber, de-seeded and diced into 1 cm pieces
1 mango, flesh diced
100 g cherry tomatoes, halved
100 g trimmed sugar snap peas, blanched
1 small red chilli, de-seeded and finely sliced (optional)
2–3 stems fresh mint leaves, torn
freshly ground black pepper

Dressing
2 tablespoons lemon (or lime) juice
2 tablespoons olive oil

1. Preheat the oven to 180°C.

2. Brush both sides of the chicken with oil and sprinkle over the curry powder. Place the chicken in an ovenproof dish and bake for 20 minutes or until cooked. Rest for 5–10 minutes then slice.

3. Meanwhile, cook the pasta in a large saucepan of boiling water until al dente, following the packet instructions for timing. Check a minute or two before the end of the cooking time. Drain in a colander and chill under running cold water to stop the cooking process. Drain well.

4. To make the dressing, combine the lemon or lime juice and oil in a small jug and whisk to combine.

5. In a serving bowl, combine the cucumber, mango, tomatoes, peas, chilli, pasta, chicken and mint leaves. Pour over the dressing, add freshly ground black pepper to taste and toss to combine.

PER SERVE
1601 kJ; 18 g fat (includes saturated fat 3 g); 4 g fibre; 18 g protein; 38 g carbohydrate

Chicken and Rice Lettuce Cups

This is a great recipe for when you have leftover chicken. Prepare it in stages: you can cook the rice and the chicken the day before and store in airtight containers in the refrigerator. Store leftover salad in an airtight container in the refrigerator for up to 1 day.

Serves 8 **Preparation time** 15 minutes
Cooking time 40 minutes + 20–30 minutes cooling time

½ cup (100 g) wild rice, rinsed and drained
1 cup (200 g) brown rice, rinsed and drained
2 cups (300 g) frozen corn and pea mix, thawed
1 (about 200 g) cooked skinless chicken breast fillet, shredded
1 green capsicum, diced
1 red capsicum, diced
1 Lebanese cucumber, de-seeded and diced
6 spring onions, finely chopped
¼ cup finely chopped fresh parsley
16 cup- or scoop-shaped iceberg or cos lettuce leaves, washed then chilled to crisp

Zesty Dressing

⅓ cup (80 ml) orange juice
¼ cup (60 ml) lemon juice
¼ cup (60 ml) olive oil
2 teaspoons finely grated ginger, or to taste
2 teaspoons lemon zest
2 teaspoons soft brown sugar, or to taste
salt and freshly ground black pepper

1. Cook the brown rice and wild rice in two separate saucepans, following the packet instructions. Fluff with a fork and set aside to cool.

2. Steam the corn and peas for 1–2 minutes or until just al dente. Rinse immediately under cold running water to cool and stop the cooking process. Drain thoroughly.

3. To make the Zesty Dressing, whisk all ingredients together in a small bowl and season to taste.

4. In a serving bowl, combine the shredded chicken with the wild rice, brown rice, corn, peas, capsicum, cucumber, spring onion and parsley. Pour over the dressing and toss well. Spoon the mixture into the lettuce cups and serve.

VARIATIONS

- Replace the chicken with flaked canned tuna or salmon, or with smoked trout.
- For a vegetarian meal, serve without the chicken.

PER SERVE – 2 LETTUCE CUPS

1150 kJ; 10 g fat (including 1.5 g saturated fat); 4 g fibre; 11 g protein; 34 g carbohydrate

---

Cooking brown rice and wild rice together

If the brown rice and wild rice you buy require the same cooking time, you can cook them together using the absorption method. In a heavybased saucepan, bring ⅓ cup wild rice and ⅔ cup brown rice to the boil in 2 cups (500 ml) water. Reduce the heat to very low, cover and simmer for 40 minutes. Remove from the heat and stand, covered, for another 20–30 minutes. Fluff with a fork.

Pistachio and Quinoa Tabbouli

Quinoa is a tiny, fast-cooking grain ideal in gluten-free dishes. It's not just low GI – it's also rich in nutrients, including protein. Enjoy this tabbouli on its own, in cos lettuce-leaf scoops, in gluten-free wraps or pitta pockets with hommous, or as a salad accompaniment to a barbecue. Store leftover salad in an airtight container in the refrigerator for up to 1 day.

Serves 6 **Preparation time** 10 minutes
Cooking time 15 minutes + resting time

1 cup (200 g) quinoa, rinsed
juice of 1 lemon, or to taste
2 tablespoons extra virgin olive oil
freshly ground black pepper
½ cup (75 g) roughly chopped pistachio nuts
1 cup chopped flat-leaf (Italian) parsley
½ cup chopped mint leaves, or to taste
1 small red (Spanish) onion, finely diced
2 large vine-ripened tomatoes, de-seeded and chopped
1 medium Lebanese cucumber, de-seeded and diced

To serve
gluten-free wraps
hommous (see Basics)

1 Place the quinoa in a medium saucepan and cover with 2 cups (500 ml) of water. Bring to the boil then reduce the heat and simmer for 10–15 minutes or until the grains are just tender and translucent and all the water is absorbed. Remove from heat and rest, covered, for 5–10 minutes. Fluff with a fork.

2 Meanwhile, whisk together the lemon juice, pepper and oil and season to taste.

3 Transfer the warm quinoa to a serving bowl with the nuts, parsley, mint, onion, tomato, cucumber and dressing. Mix well to combine. Serve in a bowl, or with gluten-free wraps and hommous, to scoop and wrap your salad, if you like.

VARIATION
- For an even more colourful salad, use red quinoa (you'll find it in health food stores) and follow the cooking times suggested on the packet.

PER SERVE OF TABBOULI ONLY
Energy 1152 kJ; 14 g fat (including 1.5 g saturated fat); 5.5 g fibre; 8 g protein; 25 g carbohydrate

Tuna Pasta Niçoise

Beans and vinaigrette-style dressing help to lower the GI of this gluten-free pasta recipe. Store leftover salad in an airtight container in the refrigerator for up to 1 day.

Serves 4 **Preparation time** 15 minutes **Cooking time** 10 minutes

- 200 g gluten-free pasta shapes
- ¼ cup (60 ml) vinaigrette dressing
- 185 g can Italian-style tuna in oil, drained and flaked
- 400 g can cannellini beans, drained and rinsed
- 1 small fennel bulb, finely sliced
- 1 small red (Spanish) onion, very finely sliced
- 3 tablespoons pitted kalamata olives
- 2 stems basil, leaves picked and roughly chopped
- 2 anchovy fillets, roughly chopped (optional)
- 1 tablespoon capers, rinsed
- 2 hard-boiled eggs, quartered
- 12 green beans, steamed 3 minutes

1 Cook the pasta in a large saucepan of boiling water, following the packet instructions and testing 1–2 minutes before end of cooking, until al dente. Drain in a colander.

2 Place in a large serving bowl. While still warm, toss with half the vinaigrette dressing.

3 Add the tuna, cannellini beans, fennel, onion, olives, basil, anchovies (if using) and capers, and toss to combine well. Top with the eggs and green beans, and sprinkle over the remaining dressing.

VARIATIONS
- Replace the tuna with the same amount of canned salmon or smoked trout.
- Replace the beans with chickpeas.
- For a vegetarian option, omit the tuna and anchovies and add 2 or 3 extra hard-boiled eggs.

PER SERVE
1706 kJ; 10 g fat (including 2 g saturated fat); 4.5 g fibre; 24 g protein; 53 g carbohydrate

Pasta salads

Pasta teams well with:

- Tomatoes, lima beans, rocket and goat's cheese tossed in a balsamic dressing
- Gluten-free ham, asparagus and baby corn tossed in a vinaigrette dressing
- Tuna, snow peas, cherry tomatoes and red kidney beans with tzatziki dressing
- Apple, celery, dried fruit and walnuts in a yoghurt dressing
- Sun-dried tomatoes, roasted capsicum strips, cannellini beans, spinach, onion and basil in a red-wine vinegar dressing
- Roasted pumpkin, pine nuts, chickpeas and rocket in a balsamic dressing, and
- Chicken, orange slices, avocado, celery and almonds in a zesty citrus dressing.

Lentil and Feta Salad

We like to use lentils that hold their shape well when cooked for salads. Good choices are French green lentils, now grown in Australia, or Puy lentils. If using brown lentils, watch the cooking time – you don't want them to get too soft for a salad. Store leftover salad in an airtight container in the refrigerator for up to 1 day.

Serves 4 **Preparation time** 15 minutes
Cooking time 25 minutes + cooling time

1 cup (200 g) French green or Puy lentils
1 red capsicum, diced
1 green capsicum, diced
1 green chilli, de-seeded and finely chopped (optional)
1 small red (Spanish) onion, finely sliced
12 cherry tomatoes, quartered
3 tablespoons finely chopped coriander
60 g feta, crumbled

Balsamic dressing
2 tablespoons olive oil
1 tablespoon balsamic vinegar
1 tablespoon lemon juice
freshly ground black pepper

1 In a medium saucepan, bring the lentils to the boil with 2 cups (500 ml) water, stirring occasionally. Reduce the heat, cover and simmer for about 20 minutes or until tender but firm to the bite. Remove from the heat, drain well and set aside to cool.

2 Meanwhile, to make the dressing, whisk all ingredients together in a small bowl.

3 In a large serving bowl, combine the lentils, capsicums, chilli (if using), onion, cherry tomatoes and coriander. Pour over the dressing and toss well to combine. Top with crumbled feta and serve.

PER SERVE
1205 kJ; 14 g fat (including 4 g saturated fat); 8.5 g fibre; 16 g protein; 22 g carbohydrate

Salad days

Did you know there's more to salad than leafy greens?

- Starting a meal with a mixed garden salad before moving on to the main course helps to fill you up and you will eat less overall.
- Eating a side salad with your meal – especially if it's a high GI meal – will help to keep your blood glucose levels under control. This is because the salad dressing acids, such as the lemon juice or vinegar, slow down stomach emptying, thereby slowing the digestion of starch in the meal you are eating.

Velvety Pumpkin Soup

This soup is one of Kate's favourites – and her clients love it too, if requests for recipe sheets are anything to go by! Purée the soup for about 10 seconds to achieve that creamy, velvety texture. Top each serving with a dollop of low fat natural yoghurt, if you like, then sprinkle over the coriander. If you make the soup the day before, store in the refrigerator in an airtight container then reheat and serve.

Serves 6 **Preparation time** 15 minutes **Cooking time** 45 minutes

2 tablespoons olive oil
2 medium onions, chopped
2.5 cm piece ginger, peeled and grated
3 teaspoons curry powder
500 g butternut pumpkin, peeled and diced
500 g orange sweet potato, peeled and diced
2 stalks celery, sliced
1 cup (250 g) split red lentils, picked over and rinsed
3 cups (750 ml) gluten-free reduced-salt chicken or vegetable stock
freshly ground black pepper
2 tablespoons finely chopped fresh coriander (or parsley), to serve

1 Heat the olive oil in a large saucepan over a medium heat. Add the onion, ginger and curry powder, reduce the heat and gently cook for 6–8 minutes or until onion is soft and golden. (Be careful it doesn't burn.)

2 Add the pumpkin, sweet potato, celery and red lentils to the pan, stir well to combine and cook a further 1 minute. Pour in the stock and 3 cups (750 ml) water, and bring to the boil. Reduce heat to low and simmer gently for 30 minutes or until the vegetables are soft. Season to taste.

3 When cool, purée the soup in batches in a food processor or blender, then reheat gently. Spoon the soup into bowls, sprinkle over the chopped coriander and serve.

PER SERVE
1059 kJ; 7 g fat (includes 1 g saturated fat); 7.5 g fibre; 12 g protein; 32 g carbohydrate,

Italian Rice and Lentil Soup

This is one of those soups your spoon almost stands up in. If that's too thick for you, just add more water. The secret of success is to make sure the onions really are soft before you proceed any further with the cooking. If you make the soup the day before, store in the refrigerator in an airtight container, then simply reheat and serve. Passata is an Italian cooking sauce. You'll find it in all good supermarkets.

Serves 6 **Preparation time** 5–10 minutes **Cooking time** 30 minutes

1 tablespoon olive oil
2 onions, finely chopped
1 clove garlic, finely chopped
40 g lean pancetta or bacon, visible fat removed, finely chopped
1 cup (250 ml) passata
3 tablespoons finely chopped parsley
2 cups (500 ml) gluten-free reduced-salt beef stock
½ cup (100 g) canaroli or arborio rice
2 x 400 g can lentils, drained and rinsed
freshly ground black pepper
¼ cup (25 g) grated Parmesan cheese, to serve

1 Heat the olive oil in a large saucepan on medium heat. Add the onion and garlic, reduce the heat, and cook for 10–12 minutes or until golden and soft. Add the pancetta and cook 1 minute more. Add the passata and parsley and cook a further 1 minute, stirring occasionally with a wooden spoon.

2 Add the stock and 3 cups (750 ml) water and bring to the boil. Reduce the heat, add the rice and simmer for 8–10 minutes. Add the lentils and cook a further 5 minutes or until the rice is cooked al dente and the lentils heated through. Season to taste.

3 Spoon into bowls, sprinkle over the Parmesan cheese and serve.

VARIATION
- For a vegetarian version, omit the pancetta and use a reduced-salt vegetable stock instead of the beef stock.

PER SERVE
Energy 1043 kJ; 6 g fat (including 1.5 g saturated fat); 3.5 g fibre; 9 g protein; 39 g carbohydrate

Prawn Laksa

Laksas are popular spicy soups that originated in Malaysia and Singapore, and now seem to be available everywhere. The thick white noodles seem to be preferred in restaurants, but we like making laksa with the thin ones and adding more vegetables. They are slightly more manageable to eat, too!

Serves 4 **Preparation time** 15 minutes **Cooking time** 10 minutes

125 g dried rice-stick noodles
4 tablespoons gluten-free red curry paste
300 g peeled and de-veined prawns
2½ cups (625 ml) gluten-free reduced-salt chicken stock
270 ml can light coconut milk
1 large carrot, cut into short thin sticks
100 g shiitake mushrooms, thinly sliced
125 g green beans, diagonally sliced
3 baby bok choy, leaves separated, washed, shredded
1 teaspoon brown sugar (optional)
1¼ cups (100 g) bean sprouts
½ cup picked coriander leaves, roughly chopped
lime wedges

1 Cook the noodles in a large saucepan of boiling water for 2 minutes or until just tender. Drain well. Divide the noodles among 4 large serving bowls.

2 Heat a large wok over high heat. Add the curry paste and prawns, and stir-fry for 3 minutes or until the prawns change colour. Add the stock and coconut milk, and bring to a simmer. Add the carrot, mushrooms and beans and cook for 2 minutes. Add the bok choy and cook for a further 1 minute or until just wilted. Remove from the heat and stir in the sugar, if using.

3 Divide the vegetables and prawns among the bowls. Ladle the broth into each bowl. Top with the bean sprouts and coriander, and serve with the lime wedges.

VARIATIONS
- Replace the prawns with 300 g skinless chicken breast, cut into thin strips.
- For a vegetarian version, replace the prawns with 300 g tofu and the chicken stock with reduced-salt vegetable stock.

PER SERVE
Energy 1502 kJ; 10 g fat (including 1.5 g saturated fat); 6.5 g fibre; 27 g protein; 37 g carbohydrate

Mexican Black Bean Soup with Corn

The great thing about cooking the low GI way is enjoying new ingredients. Black beans, also called turtle beans, have a mild earthy flavour when cooked and are widely used throughout Latin America and the Caribbean. Soaking overnight shortens the cooking time. If you make the soup the day before, store in the refrigerator in an airtight container, then simply reheat and serve the next day.

Serves 6 **Soaking time** Overnight **Preparation time** 15 minutes
Cooking time 1 hour 15 minutes

1 cup (200 g) dried black beans, soaked overnight
2 tablespoons olive oil
2 red (Spanish) onions, chopped
2 cloves garlic, crushed
2 teaspoons ground oregano
2 teaspoons ground cumin
1 red chilli, de-seeded and finely sliced, or to taste
1 red capsicum, diced
1 green capsicum, diced
2 stalks celery, sliced
2 dried bay leaves
3 cups (750 ml) gluten-free reduced-salt vegetable stock
1 cup corn kernels
2 squares of chocolate (70% cocoa) or 2 teaspoons unsweetened cocoa powder
½ cup (125 ml) orange juice
3 tablespoons finely chopped coriander (or parsley)

1 Drain the black beans from the soaking water, then rinse under cold water and drain again.

2 Heat the oil in a large, heavy-based saucepan over medium heat. Add the onion and garlic, reduce the heat and cook for 8–10 minutes or until the onion is soft and translucent. Add the oregano, cumin and chilli and cook a further 1 minute or until aromatic. Add the capsicum, celery, black beans, bay leaves, stock and 2 cups (500 ml) water and bring to the boil. Reduce the heat and simmer, uncovered, for 50 minutes. Stir in the corn kernels and continue cooking for a further 10 minutes or until the beans are tender.

3 Remove the bay leaves from the soup. Stir in the chocolate, orange juice and coriander and simmer for a further 1–2 minutes. Ladle into bowls and serve.

VARIATION

- If you want to use canned black beans (available in some health food stores), here's how. Add the canned beans and corn kernels in Step 2 with the capsicum, celery, bay leaves, stock and 2 cups (500 ml) water. Bring to the boil, then reduce the heat and simmer, uncovered, for 15 minutes. Stir in the chocolate, orange juice and coriander, and simmer for 1–2 minutes more before serving.

PER SERVE

Energy 967 kJ; 7 g fat (including 1 g saturated fat); 10.5 g fibre; 9 g protein; 32 g carbohydrate

Souped up

When you are making soup, it actually doesn't require any extra time to make a larger amount. Leftovers are ideal for lunch the next day. Or freeze the extra soup for easy meals when there's no time to cook and you need a meal in a hurry. Tasty, low GI soups to try (as well as our recipes here) include:

- Lentil and spinach
- Split pea and ham
- Long or short soup with tofu and noodles
- Bean soup
- Tomato soup, and
- Minestrone (with gluten-free pasta).

Freeze in serving portions in labelled airtight containers for up to 2 months. Thaw in the refrigerator before reheating.

Chunky Tomato Soup with Chickpeas

Moroccan spice blends are usually a combination of paprika, pepper, cassia, cumin, cloves, coriander, cardamom and nutmeg. You can add them to soups, meat and seafood dishes, or rice. Or use them to coat meat, before browning, for a casserole. This is quite a hearty soup, so add extra water or stock if you wish. If you make the soup the day before, store in the refrigerator in an airtight container then simply heat through and serve the next day.

Serves 8 **Preparation time** 10 minutes **Cooking time** 40 minutes

2 tablespoons olive oil
2 red (Spanish) onions, chopped
2 cloves garlic, crushed
2.5 cm piece ginger, peeled and grated
1 medium (250 g) sweet potato, peeled and diced
2 celery stalks, sliced
2 medium carrots, scrubbed and diced
800 g can peeled roma tomatoes, drained, chopped, and juice reserved
2 teaspoons pure floral honey
2 teaspoons Moroccan spice blend
3 cups (750 ml) gluten-free reduced-salt vegetable stock
400 g can chickpeas, rinsed and drained
¼ cup roughly chopped coriander
freshly ground black pepper

To serve

creamy style low fat natural yoghurt (allow 1 tablespoon per person)
1 tablespoon finely chopped coriander

1. Heat the oil in a large, heavy-based saucepan over medium heat. Add the onion, garlic and ginger, reduce the heat and cook for 8–10 minutes or until the onion is soft and translucent. Add the sweet potato, celery and carrots, and cook for a further 1–2 minutes, stirring occasionally.

2. Stir in the tomatoes, honey and spice mix. Pour in the stock and 3 cups (750 ml) water. Bring to the boil, then reduce the heat and simmer gently for 10–15 minutes or until the vegetables are cooked. Add the chickpeas and coriander, and cook a further 5 minutes. Season to taste and serve in bowls with a dollop of creamy yoghurt and a sprinkle of coriander.

VARIATIONS
- For a creamy tomato soup, set soup aside to cool, then blend in batches in a food processor or blender. Reheat in the saucepan and serve.
- For a stronger tomato flavour, add 1 tablespoon tomato paste at Step 2.

PER SERVE
Energy 623 kJ; 5 g fat (including 1 g saturated fat); 4.5 g fibre; 5 g protein; 17 g carbohydrate

Easy Chicken and Corn Soup

This is a quick and easy, hearty soup you can make with a takeaway chicken if you are short on time. Make sure that you buy a gluten-free chicken (without any stuffing or seasoning with gluten). Add extra water for a more liquid soup.

Serves 6 **Preparation time** 10 minutes **Cooking time** 10 minutes

200 g thick, dried rice-stick noodles
4 cups (1 litre) gluten-free reduced-salt chicken stock
2 (about 400 g) cooked skinless chicken breast fillets, shredded or finely sliced on the diagonal
1 tablespoon gluten-free soy sauce
2 cups (200 g) fresh or frozen corn kernels
50 g snow pea sprouts
2 spring onions, finely sliced

1 Cook the noodles following packet instructions. Drain and divide among 4 large serving bowls.

2 Meanwhile, in a large saucepan, bring the stock with 1 cup (250 ml) water to the boil. Reduce the heat and add the chicken, soy sauce and corn kernels. Simmer for 4 minutes or until the chicken is heated through and the corn is cooked. Stir in the snow pea sprouts and cook a further 1 minute. Ladle the soup evenly into the bowls, over the rice noodles, top with spring onion slices and serve immediately.

PER SERVE
1138 kJ; 5 g fat (including 1 g saturated fat); 2.5 g fibre; 19 g protein; 36 g carbohydrate

For that authentic Mexican flavour

You really need chipotle chillies (smoked jalapenos) canned in a thick adobo sauce for an authentic Mexican flavour. But this product is hard to come by in Australia and New Zealand. To make your own, see the recipe in Basics (page 198). You can buy chipotle chillies from specialty shops or online from Herbie's Spices (see page 248).

Chapter 11: Mains

What's for dinner? Try these main meals that are filled with flavour and bursting with nutrients along with a healthy balance of carbs, protein and the right fats.

Putting it on the plate

A basic main meal eaten by most of us – whether it's traditional Western fare, or one with Mediterranean or Asian flavours – consists of some sort of meat with vegetables, and potato, rice or pasta. There's nothing wrong with this as a starting point, but a little finetuning adjusting the proportions to match the plate model below will ensure a healthy, balanced meal.

What is the plate model? We didn't create it, but we use and recommend it because it's simple and it works. It's an easy-to-learn aid to visualising what to put on your plate. It is adaptable to different cuisines and useful when eating out.

You can use it for any serving sizes, so long as you keep the food to the proportions shown. In addition, choose foods in line with the key recommendations, such as opting for good fats, cutting back on saturated fat, and being choosy about your carbs, then you are right on track to eating a healthy diet and managing your weight.

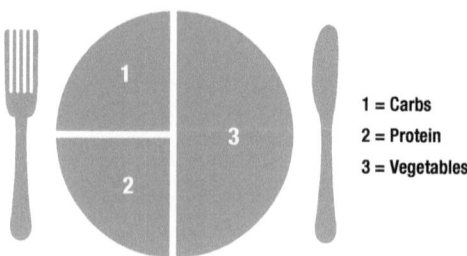

1 = Carbs
2 = Protein
3 = Vegetables

1. Carbohydrate-rich foods – bread and cereals and other starchy foods such as potatoes, legumes, sweetcorn, pasta, rice and noodles – choose low GI types
2. Protein-rich foods – meat, chicken, fish, eggs, tofu and alternatives such as legumes, milk or yoghurt
3. Vegetables

Herb Fish Parcels with Fennel, Bean and Tomato Salad

Parcels not only make fish easy to cook, they are fun to unwrap at the table, too. The parcels should cook in 15 minutes in a preheated oven, but times can vary a little depending on the thickness of the fish. The fish is cooked when it flakes easily with a fork.

Serves 4 **Preparation time** 25 minutes **Cooking time** 15 minutes

¼ cup finely chopped parsley
1 tablespoon chopped fennel leaves
2 teaspoons lemon rind
¼ teaspoon chilli flakes
1 clove garlic, crushed
1 tablespoon extra virgin olive oil
freshly ground black pepper
4 x 150 g white fish fillets

Fennel, Bean and Tomato Salad
1 fennel bulb, thinly sliced
1 punnet (250 g) cherry tomatoes, quartered
420 g can (or nearest size) four-bean mix, rinsed and drained
1 tablespoon baby capers
1 teaspoon lemon rind
¼ cup (60 ml) lemon juice
1 tablespoon extra virgin olive oil

To serve
4 steamed Carisma or Nicola potatoes or 8 small chat potatoes (optional)

1. Preheat the oven to 200°C. Tear 4 squares of baking paper (about 30 cm × 30 cm).

2. In a small bowl, combine the parsley, fennel leaves, lemon rind, chilli, garlic and oil, and season to taste with freshly ground black pepper.

3. Place a piece of fish on each square of baking paper and spread the herb mix evenly over each. Fold and wrap the baking paper securely to enclose the fish. Arrange the parcels on a baking tray and bake for 15 minutes.

4. To make the salad, combine the fennel, tomatoes, beans, capers and lemon rind in a serving bowl. Whisk together the lemon juice and oil in a small bowl and toss through salad.

5. Place a fish parcel on each plate with a generous scoop or two of salad alongside and a steamed potato for extra carbs if you wish.

PER SERVE WITHOUT POTATO
1366 kJ; 13 g fat (including 2.5 g saturated fat); 7 g fibre; 36 g protein; 13 g carbohydrate

Barbecued Lemon Chicken Skewers

We've allowed an hour to marinate the chicken, but if you have the time, leave it a little longer to absorb the flavours of the marinade. The skewer enters the meat 3–4 times, like a needle threading through cloth.

Serves 4 **Preparation time** 25 minutes **Marinating time** 1 hour
Cooking time 30 minutes + standing time

600 g skinless chicken breasts (2 large)

Marinade
1 teaspoon finely grated lemon rind
½ cup (125 ml) lemon juice
1 teaspoon chopped fresh rosemary
3 teaspoons Dijon mustard
2 cloves garlic, crushed
1 tablespoon olive oil

Bean and Asparagus Pilaf
1 bunch asparagus, cut into 2 cm pieces
120 g green beans, trimmed and cut into 2 cm pieces
2 teaspoons olive oil
1 onion, chopped
1 clove garlic, crushed
1 cup (200 g) basmati rice
2 cups (500 ml) gluten-free, reduced-salt chicken stock
2 tablespoons chopped parsley

To serve
green salad with vinaigrette dressing

1 Soak 12 wooden skewers in water for 30 minutes.

2 Meanwhile, slice each chicken breast into 6 × 1 cm thick, long slices. You should have 12 long slices. Place 4 pieces on a sheet of plastic wrap, and cover with another sheet of plastic wrap. Use a rolling pin or mallet to flatten the pieces to about ½ cm thick. Repeat with the remaining slices.

3 To make the marinade, combine all the ingredients in a medium bowl. Reserve ¼ cup (60 ml) of the mixture and set aside.

4 Add the chicken to remaining marinade in the bowl and chill in the refrigerator for 1 hour.

5 Meanwhile, to make the pilaf, steam the asparagus and beans for 2–3 minutes or until tender. Drain, rinse under cold water and set aside.

6 Heat the oil in a medium saucepan. Add the onion and cook for 3–4 minutes or until soft and golden. Add the garlic and rice, and cook for a further 1 minute, stirring. Add the stock, bring to the boil, then reduce the heat to low and simmer, covered, for 15 minutes. Stand for 5 minutes. Stir through the beans, asparagus, parsley and reserved marinade. Set aside, keeping warm.

7 Thread the chicken onto the skewers. Heat the barbecue or chargrill and cook chicken each side for 2 minutes or until golden and cooked through.

8 To serve, spoon about ½ cup pilaf onto each plate, top with chicken and serve with the salad.

PER SERVE WITHOUT SALAD
2029 kJ; 16 g fat (including 3.5 g saturated fat); 2.5 g fibre; 38 g protein; 46 g carbohydrate

Cranberry Chicken with Quinoa

We have allowed for 1 small chicken breast per person. But eat to appetite. If you have leftovers, this dish is delicious the next day – hot or cold.

Serves 4 **Preparation time** 30 minutes **Cooking time** 30 minutes

¼ cup (about ½ small) coarsely grated green apple
¼ cup (40 g) craisins (dried cranberries)
2 tablespoons finely chopped walnuts
1 finely chopped spring onion
1 tablespoon finely chopped parsley
4 small (800 g) skinless chicken breasts
1 red (Spanish) onion, sliced into thin wedges
a little olive oil
freshly ground black pepper
½ cup (125 ml) gluten-free, reduced-salt chicken stock
⅓ cup (80 ml) white wine

Quinoa Pilaf

2 teaspoons olive oil
1 small red (Spanish) onion, chopped
1 cup (200 g) quinoa, washed and drained
2 teaspoons chopped sage
2 cups (500 ml) gluten-free reduced-salt chicken stock
1 tablespoon chopped parsley

To serve

steamed beans and carrots

1. Preheat the oven to 200°C.

2. Combine apple, craisins, walnuts, spring onion and parsley in a bowl.

3. Cut a deep slit (not all the way through) along the length of each chicken breast and spread with the apple filling. Use toothpicks to secure the openings.

4. Place the chicken in an ovenproof baking dish and surround with the onion wedges. Brush the chicken with olive oil and grind some pepper over it. Combine the stock and wine in a small jug and pour over the chicken. Bake for 25–30 minutes or until chicken is cooked through.

5. Meanwhile, to make the quinoa pilaf, heat the oil in a medium-sized saucepan and add the onion. Cook for 3–4 minutes or until soft and golden (don't let the onion burn). Add the quinoa and sage, stir, add the stock and bring to the boil. Reduce the heat, cover and simmer for 12–15 minutes. Stand for 5 minutes and then fluff the quinoa with a fork. Stir through the parsley.

6. Remove toothpicks from the chicken and slice each breast diagonally into 2 pieces.

7 To serve, spoon about ½ cup quinoa pilaf onto each plate, top with 1–2 slices of chicken and drizzle over a little of the cooking sauce. Serve with beans and carrots.

PER SERVE WITH BEANS AND CARROTS
2631 kJ; 22 g fat (including 4.5 g saturated fat); 8.7 g fibre; 52 g protein; 48 g carbohydrate

Quick and easy quinoa

Quinoa (pronounced keen-wah) is a small, round, quick-cooking grain somewhat similar in colour to sesame seeds. It's a nutritional powerpack – an excellent source of low GI carbs (GI 51), fibre and protein, and rich in B vitamins and minerals including iron, phosphorus, magnesium and zinc. You can buy quinoa flakes and quinoa flour, but these products haven't been GI tested yet. Health and organic food stores and larger supermarkets are the best places to shop for quinoa. You may find it's a little more expensive than other grains. It cooks in about 10–15 minutes (follow the packet instructions) and has a light, chewy texture and slightly nutty flavour.

- Substitute quinoa for rice or other grains for gluten-free soups, stuffed vegetables, salads, stews and even in a 'rice' pudding or porridge.
- To serve four as a side dish, rinse 1 cup of quinoa. Drain, place the grains in a medium-sized pot with 2 cups of water and bring to the boil. Reduce heat, cover and leave to barely simmer until all the water has been absorbed.
- For a richer flavour, toast quinoa (but don't let it burn) in a dry pan for a minute or two before cooking as above.

Easy Tuna Bake

Every family seems to have its own version of a comforting tuna bake. The perfect meal on a wintry evening when everyone is a bit tired after a long day. Make it with low GI gluten-free pasta if you can. If it's not available, don't worry as we have added lots of other low GI ingredients like milk, corn and peas to reduce the GI of this tasty dish.

Serves 4 **Preparation time** 25 minutes **Cooking time** 55 minutes

olive oil spray
1 cup (80 g) gluten-free pasta spirals (or small shapes like macaroni)
425 g can tuna in oil, drained, flaked
1 small red capsicum, diced
3 spring onions, sliced
⅓ cup (45 g) gluten-free cornflour
2 cups (500 ml) reduced-fat milk
⅓ cup (30 g) finely grated Parmesan cheese
3 tablespoons finely chopped parsley
freshly ground black pepper
2 cups (300 g) frozen corn and pea mix
1 tablespoon Dijon mustard

Topping
⅔ cup fresh gluten-free low GI breadcrumbs
½ teaspoon paprika
10 g reduced-fat margarine

1 Preheat the oven to 180°C. Spray a 2-litre capacity baking dish with olive oil spray.

2 Cook the pasta according to the directions on the packet until only just al dente (remember you are going to be baking it as well), drain, cover and set aside.

3 In a large bowl combine the tuna, capsicum and spring onions.

4 Stir the cornflour with a little of the milk in a small jug until it dissolves. Heat the remaining milk in a large saucepan and bring just to the boil. Add the cornflour mix and stir until the mixture boils, then reduce the heat to low and simmer for 1 minute while continuing to stir. Turn off the heat and stir through the cheese, parsley and freshly ground black pepper.

5 Add the tuna mix to the mixture in the saucepan along with the corn and pea mix, mustard and the pasta. Combine well. Spoon the mixture into the prepared baking dish and smooth the top.

6 For the topping, combine breadcrumbs and paprika and rub in margarine. Sprinkle this evenly over the tuna mixture. Bake in the oven for 40 minutes or until the top is golden and crunchy. Serve with a garden salad

VARIATIONS
- Replace the frozen pea and corn mix with 310 g can corn, drained, and 1 cup frozen peas.
- To make the tuna bake more child-friendly for littlies, substitute the breadcrumb topping with a mix of crushed gluten-free snack crisps, such as Chick Pea Chips, and a sprinkle of reduced-fat cheddar cheese.

PER SERVE
2364 kJ; 22 g fat (including 5.5 g saturated fat); 6.5 g fibre; 40 g protein; 49 g carbohydrate

Fruity Lamb Casserole

When you are making a casserole, after the meat is browned, the pan is usually 'deglazed'. This means you add liquid such as wine or stock to loosen and dissolve the brown bits on the base formed during cooking. This way you enjoy all the flavour.

Serves 4 **Preparation time** 20 minutes **Cooking time** 1½ hours

1 tablespoon olive oil
500 g trimmed diced shoulder lamb
1 onion, chopped
¼ cup (60 ml) red wine
2 cloves garlic, crushed
2 tablespoons chermoula spice mix
2 cups (500 ml) gluten-free reduced-salt chicken stock
200 g sweet potato, peeled and chopped into 2 cm chunks
1 large parsnip, peeled and chopped into 1 cm chunks
2 small zucchinis, sliced into 2 cm chunks
80 g dried apricots
80 g pitted prunes
40 g currants
2 tablespoons chopped parsley

Mint Yoghurt
200 g tub low fat plain yoghurt
1 tablespoon finely chopped mint
1 teaspoon finely grated lemon zest
freshly ground black pepper

To serve
steamed broccolini

1 Heat the oil in a large saucepan. Add half the lamb pieces, and brown on all sides for about 3 minutes. Spoon into a dish and set aside. Repeat with the remaining lamb and keep warm.

2 To deglaze the pan, add the onion and wine and let it cook for 3–4 minutes on a low heat. Add the garlic and chermoula spice mix and cook for 1 minute more, stirring regularly.

3 Return the meat to the pan with the stock, stir to combine and bring to the boil. Reduce the heat to low, cover and simmer gently for 50 minutes. Add the sweet potato, parsnip, zucchinis, dried apricots, pitted prunes and currants, and bring back to the boil. Reduce the heat to low, cover and simmer for 20 minutes more. Remove the lid and cook, uncovered, for 5 minutes. Stir in parsley.

4 To make the Mint Yoghurt, combine the yoghurt, mint and lemon zest in a small serving bowl and season to taste.

5 Serve the casserole topped with a dollop of Mint Yoghurt and lots of steamed broccolini or your favourite green vegetable alongside.

PER SERVE WITH YOGHURT AND BROCCOLINI
1915 kJ; 12 g fat (including 4 g saturated fat); 10.5 g fibre; 36 g protein; 42 g carbohydrate

Greek-style Beef Skewers

Allow 4 pieces of meat, 5 pieces of capsicum and 2 pieces of mushroom per skewer.

Serves 4 **Preparation time** 30 minutes **Marinating time** 30 minutes **Cooking time** 10 minutes

400 g lean beef rump, cut into 2–3 cm cubes
1 small red capsicum, cut into 2–3 cm pieces
1 small green capsicum, cut into 2–3 cm pieces
8 button mushrooms, cut in half

Herb Rub

1 tablespoon dried oregano
2 teaspoons dried mint
3 teaspoons lemon zest
3 cloves garlic, crushed
1½ tablespoons olive oil
2 tablespoons lemon juice

Tomato and Bean Salad

3 small tomatoes, quartered
2 Lebanese cucumbers, sliced
1 small red (Spanish) onion, halved and thinly sliced
440 g can butter beans, drained and rinsed
3 tablespoons pitted kalamata olives
2 tablespoons extra virgin olive oil
2 tablespoons lemon juice
1 tablespoon white wine vinegar
½ teaspoon dried oregano

To serve

8 steamed small chat or 4 Carisma or Nicola potatoes or gluten-free wraps

1. Place 8 long wooden skewers in water and set aside to soak for 30 minutes.

2. Meanwhile, to make the Herb Rub, combine the dried oregano, dried mint, lemon zest, garlic, olive oil and lemon juice in a medium bowl. Add the beef and mix well so that all the meat is thoroughly coated. Cover and set aside to marinate in the refrigerator for 30 minutes, or longer if time permits.

3. To make the Tomato and Bean Salad, combine the tomatoes, cucumber, onion, beans and olives in a serving bowl. Whisk together the oil, lemon juice, vinegar and oregano in a small bowl. Pour over the salad and toss well.

4. Thread each skewer with beef cubes, capsicum and mushrooms, alternating each ingredient and starting with capsicum.

5. Heat a chargrill or barbecue on medium–high heat and brush over a little oil. Cook the kebabs, turning frequently, for 8 minutes or until meat is done to your liking. Serve immediately with salad and with 1–2 wraps or potatoes per person if you wish.

PER SERVE WITH GLUTEN-FREE WRAPS
2068 kJ; 24 g fat (including 5 g saturated fat); 5.5 g fibre; 28 g protein; 38 g carbohydrate

Lamb Curry with Spinach Rice Pilaf

We used Herbie's Mild Curry Powder in this recipe. If you can't find it locally, you can make your own blend. It is worth the effort for the flavour and aroma, without the heat. See Basics (page 199).

Serves 4 **Preparation time** 25 minutes **Cooking time** 35 minutes

1½ tablespoons gluten-free curry powder
400 g lamb backstrap, diced into 2–3 cm pieces
1 tablespoon canola oil
1 onion, chopped
2 cloves garlic, crushed
1 teaspoon grated ginger
2 carrots, chopped into 2 cm chunks
400 g can chopped tomatoes
2 cups cauliflower florets
¾ cup (190 ml) gluten-free reduced-salt chicken stock
1 cup (150 g) frozen green peas

Spinach Rice Pilaf

1 tablespoon canola oil
1 onion, chopped
½ cup (100 g) basmati or Moolgiri rice
1 cup (250 ml) gluten-free reduced-salt chicken stock
1 bay leaf
400 g can lentils, drained and rinsed
60 g baby spinach leaves

1 Sprinkle 2 teaspoons of the curry powder over the lamb to coat the pieces lightly. Heat 2 teaspoons of the oil in a large, heavy-based saucepan, add the lamb and brown both sides for 2–3 minutes in 2 batches. Spoon the browned meat into a dish, cover and set aside, keeping warm.

2 Heat the remaining oil in the pan. Add the onion and cook for 3–4 minutes until soft and golden. Add the garlic, ginger, remaining curry powder and carrots, and cook, stirring, for 1 minute.

3 Return the meat to the pan with the tomatoes, cauliflower and stock. Bring to the boil, then reduce the heat to low, cover, and simmer gently for 20 minutes. Add the peas and cook for another 2 minutes.

4 Meanwhile, to make the rice pilaf, heat the oil in a medium-sized saucepan. Add the onion and cook for 3–4 minutes until soft and golden. Add the rice and cook, stirring, for another 1 minute. Add the stock and bay leaf and bring to the boil. Reduce the heat to low, cover, and simmer very gently for 15 minutes.

5 Stir in the lentils, heat through, and then stir through the spinach.

6 To serve, spoon a little pilaf on each plate and top with the curry.

VARIATION

- To make Curried Spinach Rice Pilaf, add 1 teaspoon curry powder to the pan when adding the rice.

PER SERVE
1887 kJ; 17 g fat (including 4 g saturated fat); 9 g fibre; 31 g protein; 38 g carbohydrate

Pork with Glazed Apple and Cannellini Mash

Cloudy apple juice is a wonderful ingredient in savoury dishes and baking, as it adds a touch of sweetness. We now know that cloudy apple juice has almost four times more antioxidants than clear apple juice because it retains its healthy pulp, with all the fibre.

Serves 4 **Preparation time** 15 minutes **Marinating time** 30 minutes **Cooking time** 25 minutes

¼ cup (60 ml) unsweetened cloudy apple juice
2 teaspoons gluten-free reduced-salt tamari
2 teaspoons maple syrup
¼ teaspoon ground fennel
freshly ground black pepper
2 x 300 g pork fillets
1 tablespoon olive oil
3 green apples, quartered, cored and sliced into thick wedges
1–2 tablespoons gluten-free, reduced-salt chicken stock

Cannellini Mash

2 cups (270 g) frozen broad beans
400 g can cannellini beans, drained and rinsed
1 teaspoon reduced-fat margarine
¼ teaspoon ground fennel, optional

To serve

steamed green beans
steamed, scrubbed baby carrots

1. Preheat the oven to 200°C. Line an ovenproof baking tray with baking paper.

2. In a small bowl, combine the apple juice, tamari, maple syrup and fennel, and season with pepper. Place the pork fillets in a dish long enough to fit them, brush well with the apple juice mixture, cover and marinate in the refrigerator for 30 minutes, or longer if time permits.

3. To make the Cannellini Mash, bring a saucepan of water to the boil, add the broad beans and cook for 3 minutes. Drain and refresh under cold running water. When cool enough to handle, peel the skin from the beans. Combine the broad beans with the cannellini beans in a medium bowl and mash with a fork (it should have some texture). Set aside.

4. In a large frying pan, heat 2 teaspoons of oil, add the pork fillets (reserving the marinade) and cook for 3–4 minutes, turning to make sure they are browned all over. Transfer to the baking tray and roast for 15 minutes. Cover with foil and set aside to rest.

5 Meanwhile, heat the remaining oil in the same frying pan. Add the apples and cook, stirring occasionally, for 12 minutes or until just tender. If the apples begin to stick, add 1–2 tablespoons of chicken stock. When the apples are cooked, add the reserved marinade. Let it bubble for a few seconds until it turns syrupy and then remove pan from heat and set aside.

6 To heat the Cannellini Mash, melt the margarine in a small saucepan. Add the mash and ground fennel, if using, and stir until heated through.

7 To serve, spoon a little mash on each plate, slice the pork on the diagonal, top with the apple and drizzle over the syrupy juices. Serve with beans and carrots or your favourite vegetables.

PER SERVE WITH BEANS AND CARROTS
1824 kJ; 10 g fat (including 2 g saturated fat); 9 g fibre; 45 g protein; 38 g carbohydrate

Pork, Bok Choy and Noodle Stir-Fry

This stir-fry really is a one-pot wonder. Not only do you use one frying pan or wok, but at the end you have a nourishing and satisfying meal with lots of vegetables – all in one bowl. Older children can help with the slicing.

Serves 4 **Preparation time** 20 minutes **Cooking time** 15 minutes

200 g dry rice noodles
2 tablespoons gluten-free reduced-salt tamari
2 tablespoons gluten-free sweet chilli sauce
1 teaspoon sesame oil
1 tablespoon canola oil
500 g pork fillet, sliced thinly
1 red (Spanish) onion, sliced into thin wedges
2 teaspoons finely grated fresh ginger
1 red capsicum, sliced into thin strips
115 g (or use nearest sized punnet) baby corn, sliced in half lengthwise
150 g snow peas, trimmed, sliced diagonally in half
1 bunch baby bok choy, trimmed, halved at stem joint, stem bases removed, leaves and stems sliced
⅓ cup (50 g) toasted cashews, chopped roughly

1 Prepare the noodles according to packet directions, drain and set aside.

2 In a small bowl, combine the tamari, sweet chilli sauce and sesame oil and set aside.

3 In a large frying pan or wok, heat 2 teaspoons of canola oil. Add half the pork strips and stir-fry for 1–2 minutes or until just cooked. Spoon into a heatproof bowl and set aside. Repeat with the remaining pork.

4 Heat the remaining oil in the pan over medium–high heat. Add the onion and stir-fry for 2 minutes. Add the ginger, capsicum and corn, and stir-fry for about 1 minute. Add the snow peas and bok choy stems, and stir-fry for a further 1 minute. (Add a little water or gluten-free reduced-salt chicken stock to pan, if it starts to stick.)

5 Return the pork to the pan with tamari mix, bok choy leaves and the noodles. Toss until well combined and heated through.

6 Spoon into serving bowls and serve sprinkled with cashew nuts.

VARIATION
- To make a vegetarian version, Tofu, Bok Choy and Noodle Stir Fry, replace the pork with 300 g firm tofu, drained and cut into 2 cm cubes.

PER SERVE
1984 kJ; 15 g fat (including 2.5 g saturated fat); 5 g fibre; 36 g protein; 45 g carbohydrate

Oodles of noodles

Gluten-free noodles (rice, buckwheat or bean thread) are a great standby for quick meals. Served with fish, chicken, tofu or lean meat and plenty of vegetables, a soup, salad or stir-fry based on noodles gives you a healthy balance of smart carbs, fats and proteins plus some fibre and essential vitamins and minerals. To cook, follow the instructions on the packet as times vary depending on types and thickness. Some noodles only need swirling under running warm water to separate, or soaking in hot (but not boiling) water to soften before you serve them or add to stir-fries. Others need to be boiled. Like pasta, they are usually best just tender, almost al dente, so keep an eye on the clock.

As it's all too easy to slurp, gulp, twirl and overeat noodles, keep those portion sizes moderate. While they are a low to moderate GI choice themselves, eating a huge amount will have a marked effect on your blood glucose. Instead of piling your plate with noodles, serve plenty of vegetables – a cup of noodles combined with lots of mixed vegetables can turn into three cups of a noodle-based meal and fit into any adult's or teenager's daily diet. Remember when planning meals that the sauces you serve with noodles and how you cook them (if they are crisp they are deep-fried) can provide a lot more kilojoules than the noodles themselves.

Pumpkin, Ricotta and Lentil Lasagne

A lasagne can seem like a lot of effort when you are pressed for time. But it's such a favourite on wintry evenings and a great (and economical) way to feed a hungry crowd. To save time, you can make the lentil sauce and bake the pumpkin the night before, so that all you need to do the next day is assemble the dish and pop it in the oven.

Serves: 6–8 **Preparation time** 35 minutes **Cooking time** 1¾ hours

olive oil spray
400 g peeled butternut pumpkin, sliced thinly
1 tablespoon olive oil
2 teaspoons chopped fresh rosemary
freshly ground black pepper
1 large onion, chopped
1 carrot, halved lengthwise, then thinly sliced
2 cloves garlic, crushed
2 tablespoons tomato paste
400 g can chopped tomatoes
400 g can lentils, drained and rinsed
½ teaspoon sugar
80 g baby spinach leaves
¼ cup chopped fresh parsley
500 g low fat ricotta cheese
1 egg
½ cup (125 ml) skim milk
½ cup (50 g) finely grated Parmesan cheese
200 g packet gluten-free lasagne sheets

To serve

green, mixed leaf salad with a vinaigrette dressing

1 Preheat the oven to 200°C. Line a baking tray with baking paper. Grease a 20 cm × 30 cm × 5 cm deep baking dish with olive oil spray.

2 In a medium bowl, toss the pumpkin with 2 teaspoons oil, rosemary and freshly ground black pepper. Place the well-coated pumpkin slices on the tray and bake for 15–18 minutes or until cooked. Set aside.

3 In a medium, heavy-based saucepan, heat the remaining oil. Add the onion and carrot, and cook, stirring occasionally, for 5 minutes. Add the garlic, tomato paste and tomatoes, bring to the boil, then reduce heat to low and simmer gently for 5 minutes. Add the lentils and sugar and cook for 5 minutes or until the carrot is tender. Remove from the heat and stir in the spinach and parsley.

4 In a small bowl, combine the ricotta, egg, milk and ¼ cup of the Parmesan cheese. Season with pepper and mix together well.

5 Spoon ⅔ cup of the lentil sauce over the base of the baking dish and spread evenly. Lay 3 lasagne sheets evenly over this. Spread 1 cup of lentil sauce over the lasagne sheets, then half the pumpkin and then ⅓ of the ricotta mix. Repeat layering with the lasagne sheets, 1 cup of the lentil sauce, the remaining pumpkin and then ⅓ of the ricotta mix. (You may need to break up some of the lasagne sheets to fit over the sauce). Lay the remaining lasagne sheets over the top. Top with the remaining lentil mix and then the ricotta mix. Sprinkle with the remaining Parmesan cheese.

6 Cover the dish with foil and bake for 30 minutes. Uncover and bake for another 30–35 minutes or until top is golden. Cut into 8 even portions and serve with lots of crispy green salad.

PER SERVE FOR 8 SERVES WITHOUT SALAD
1208 kJ; 11 g fat (including 5.5 g saturated fat); 3 g fibre; 16 g protein; 30 g carbohydrate

Vegetarian Pad Thai

The secret for successful Asian cooking is to have all the ingredients prepared and ready in front of you before you start cooking.

Serves 4 **Preparation time** 25 minutes **Marinating time** 30 minutes
Cooking time 15 minutes + standing time

300 g firm tofu, drained, cut into cubes
¼ cup (60 ml) gluten-free reduced-salt tamari
2 teaspoons gluten-free plum sauce
1 clove garlic, crushed
1 teaspoon finely grated fresh ginger
2 tablespoons lime juice
1 teaspoon caster sugar
200 g gluten-free dried rice-stick noodles
1 tablespoon canola oil
1 onion, cut into thin wedges
1 long red chilli, de-seeded, cut into thin strips
1 red capsicum, thinly sliced
100 g bean sprouts, trimmed
¼ cup chopped garlic chives
¼ cup chopped coriander
1 spring onion, thinly sliced

To serve

¼ cup (35 g) chopped toasted cashews
lime wedges

1 Place the tofu in a shallow, non-metallic dish. In a small bowl, combine 2 tablespoons of the tamari with the plum sauce, garlic and ginger. Pour the tamari marinade over the tofu, cover and set aside in the refrigerator to marinate for at least 30 minutes.

2 Place the remaining tamari, lime juice and sugar in a small bowl and stir with a fork to combine. Set aside.

3 Place the noodles in a large heatproof bowl and pour over enough boiling water to cover. Stand for 5 minutes then drain and set aside.

4 Heat half the oil in a wok over high heat. With a slotted spoon, add the tofu in batches and cook for 2–3 minutes or until golden-brown. Remove from the wok and set aside in a clean bowl. Reserve any remaining tofu marinade.

5 Add the remaining oil to the wok with the onion and chilli, and stir-fry for 2 minutes. Add the capsicum and bean sprouts and stir-fry for 1 minute more.

6 Add the noodles and lime juice mixture to the wok and toss gently over high heat for 2 minutes or until noodles are coated in the sauce and heated through. Return the tofu to the wok with the reserved tofu marinade, garlic chives, coriander and spring onion, and cook for 1 minute more.

7 Spoon the Pad Thai into bowls and serve topped with cashews and accompanied by lime wedges.

PER SERVE
1547 kJ; 15 g fat (including 2 g saturated fat); 4 g fibre; 16 g protein; 40 g carbohydrate

Moroccan Seafood Stew

We used a gluten-free seafood mix from a seafood store (rather than a frozen mix).

Serves 4 **Preparation time** 20 minutes **Cooking time** 20 minutes

Ingredients:
- 2 teaspoons olive oil
- 1 onion, chopped
- 1 fennel bulb, sliced
- 1 carrot, diced
- 2 cloves garlic, crushed
- 2 long red chillies, de-seeded and finely chopped
- 2 teaspoons ground cumin
- 2 teaspoons ground coriander
- ¼ teaspoon cinnamon
- 1 cup (250 ml) water or gluten-free reduced-salt fish stock
- 500 g gluten-free seafood mix
- 2 tomatoes, diced
- 120 g sugar snap peas, cut in half
- 400 g can chickpeas, drained and rinsed
- 30 g rocket
- 30 g spinach
- 2 tablespoons chopped coriander
- lemon wedges

1 Heat the oil in a large, heavy-based saucepan. Add the onion and cook for 2–3 minutes. Add the fennel, carrot, garlic, chilli and spices, and cook for 1 minute more. Gradually add the stock, stirring, and then bring to the boil. Reduce the heat to low and simmer for 10 minutes, stirring occasionally.

2 Add the seafood mix and tomatoes, and cook for 3 minutes or until seafood has just cooked. In the last minute, add sugar snap peas. Then stir through chickpeas, rocket and spinach until heated through. Stir in the coriander.

3 Ladle the stew into bowls and serve with lemon wedges alongside.

PER SERVING
1284 kJ; 8 g fat (including 1.5 g saturated fat); 8 g fibre; 38 g protein; 18 g carbohydrate

Chapter 12: Desserts

Sweet endings like these desserts can help you increase your intake of deliciously healthy, low GI fruits and low fat dairy foods. Of course, some of them are to keep for very special occasions!

Berry and Pear Cobbler

This is a traditional winter warmer. Serve with a dollop of low fat ice-cream or vanilla yoghurt for an old-fashioned treat.

Serves 4 **Preparation time** 20 minutes
Cooking time 30–35 minutes + cooling time

300 g frozen mixed berries
410 g can pears in natural juice, drained and sliced
2 teaspoons caster sugar

Topping
½ cup (70 g) brown rice flour
⅓ cup (45 g) gluten-free cornflour
2 teaspoons gluten-free baking powder
½ teaspoon xanthan gum
¼ cup (55 g) caster sugar
2 teaspoons psyllium husks
30 g reduced-fat margarine
¼ cup (60 ml) buttermilk
1 teaspoon vanilla essence
2 tablespoons almond meal

To serve
low fat ice-cream or vanilla yoghurt

1. Preheat the oven to 180°C. Mix together the berries, pear slices and sugar, and spoon into a 1½-litre-capacity (5–6 cm high) ovenproof dish.

2. To make the topping, sift the flours, baking powder and xanthan gum into a medium-sized bowl, stir to combine the mixture and then sift again into another bowl. Stir in the sugar and psyllium husks. Rub the margarine into the flour mix until it resembles breadcrumbs.

3. Combine the buttermilk and vanilla essence in a small jug. Pour into the flour mix and mix with a palette knife, using a cutting motion, until the mixture comes together. Knead quickly and lightly for a few seconds to make a smooth dough.

4. Divide the dough into 8 small portions. Form each portion into a ball and then flatten slightly to make a 'scone' shape.

5. Sprinkle the almond meal evenly over the fruit mix. Place the dough shapes over the top. (It won't cover the fruit completely – this doesn't matter, as the fruit bubbles up around the scones). Bake for 30–35 minutes or until the top is a light golden-brown. Stand for 5 minutes before serving with ice-cream or yoghurt.

PER SERVE WITHOUT ICE-CREAM
1193 kJ; 7 g fat (including 1 g saturated fat); 5 g fibre; 5 g protein; 50 g carbohydrate

Berry Yoghurt Delight

This is the perfect dessert when berries are in season. Frozen berries are a good substitute when they're not in season, but you need to allow a little extra thawing time in Step 1. We originally intended to serve this dessert with meringues, but Diane tested it with amaretti biscuits and it was so delicious and so effortless we changed our minds! However, the meringue recipe follows, just in case you would like to try the alternative.

Serves 4 **Preparation time** 15 minutes

200 g (1 punnet) strawberries
150 g (1 punnet) blueberries or raspberries
1 tablespoon runny honey
300 g low fat plain yoghurt
1½ tablespoons caster sugar
1 teaspoon finely grated lime zest
8 (about 32 g) gluten-free amaretti biscuits, crushed lightly

1. Wash, dry and hull the strawberries. Slice them and combine in a bowl with the blueberries and honey. Whisk the yoghurt with the sugar and lime zest. Taste for sweetness and add a little more sugar if needed.

2. Divide the berries evenly among 4 dessert dishes, spoon over 2–3 tablespoons of yoghurt mixture, top with a sprinkling of crushed amaretti biscuits and serve immediately.

PER SERVE
648 kJ; 1 g fat (negligible saturated fat); 2.5 g fibre; 6 g protein; 29 g carbohydrate

Meringues

Makes 24 **Preparation time** 15 minutes
Cooking time 1 hour + 2 hours cooling time

2 egg whites
½ cup (110 g) caster sugar
½ teaspoon vanilla essence
¼ cup (20 g) toasted almond flakes

1. Preheat the oven to 120°C. Line 2 baking trays with baking paper.

2. In a large bowl, beat the egg whites until soft peaks form. Gradually add the sugar, beating after each addition. Beat for 1 extra minute. Fold in the vanilla essence and almonds.

3. Place tablespoons of the mixture 3–4 cm apart on the trays. Bake for 1 hour. Leave in the oven to cool with the door ajar. Store the cool meringues in an airtight container.

PER MERINGUE
107 kJ; 1 g fat (no saturated fat); 0 g fibre; 0.5 g protein; 4 g carbohydrate

Chocolate Mousse

This is the simplest and most decadent-tasting chocolate mousse recipe you'll ever make. It's foolproof, made in minutes, and just needs about 2 hours chilling to set before serving. It has lots of saturated fat, so do keep it for a very special treat only.

Serves 4 **Preparation time** 5 minutes
Cooking time 5 minutes + cooling time **Chilling time** 2 hours

100 g dark chocolate (63% cocoa), roughly chopped
⅓ cup (80 ml) reduced-fat evaporated milk
½ teaspoon vanilla extract
200 g reduced-fat, honey-flavoured yoghurt

1. Place the chocolate and milk in a heatproof bowl. Place over a saucepan of simmering water and stir until chocolate has melted and mixture is smooth.

2. Remove from heat and add vanilla extract. Set aside to cool for 5 minutes, then add yoghurt and whisk until smooth.

3. Pour mixture into 4 × ½-cup-capacity serving glasses and set in the refrigerator for 2 hours before serving.

PER SERVE
4 serves: 777 kJ; 8 g fat (including 7.5 g saturated fat); 1 g fibre; 5 g protein; 23 g carbohydrate
6 serves: 518 kJ; 5 g fat (including 5 g saturated fat); 1 g fibre; 4 g protein; 16 g carbohydrate

Passionfruit Banana Cups

Serves 2 **Preparation time** 5 minutes

200 g low fat plain yoghurt
1 large banana (just ripe), peeled and sliced
2 passionfruit
2 Coconut and Lime Macaroons (see page 187)

1. Spoon the yoghurt evenly into 2 small cups. Divide the banana between the cups and top with the passionfruit. Serve with a Coconut and Lime Macaroon alongside.

VARIATION

- To make Mango Maple Cups, replace the banana with 1 mango. To dice the mango, remove mango cheeks, one at a time, with a sharp knife by slicing as close to the stone as possible. In each cheek, score 3–4 lines vertically and 3–4 lines horizontally to form a hatched pattern. (Take care not to cut through the skin.) Holding both edges of the fruit firmly, turn each cheek inside out. The cubes can then be sliced off. Mix 1 tablespoon maple syrup into the yoghurt.

PER SERVE WITHOUT MACAROON
503 kJ; 0.5 g fat (negligible saturated fat); 4 g fibre; 7 g protein; 19 g carbohydrate

Coconut and Lime Macaroons

Makes 30 **Preparation time** 20 minutes **Cooking time** 35 minutes
Cooling time 2 hours

1 cup (65 g) shredded coconut
2 egg whites
½ cup (110 g) sugar
¼ cup (30 g) almond meal
1 teaspoon finely grated lime rind

1 Preheat oven to 170°C. Line 2 baking trays with baking paper.

2 Place the coconut on a third baking tray and toast in the oven, stirring once, for 3–4 minutes or until golden. Set aside to cool. Reduce the oven temperature to 150°C.

3 In a medium bowl, beat the egg whites with an electric beater until soft peaks form. Gradually add the sugar, about a teaspoon at a time, and continue beating with each addition and then beat for a further minute. Fold through the coconut, almond meal and lime rind with a metal spoon until just combined.

4 Spoon tablespoons of the mixture 3–4 cm apart on the lined trays. Bake in the oven for 20 minutes, swap trays around, and then cook for a further 10 minutes. Leave trays in oven, with the door ajar, to cool.

PER MACAROON
145 kJ; 2 g fat (including 1.5 g saturated fat); 0.5 g fibre; 0.5 g protein; 4 g carbohydrate

Chocolate Almond Cake

Have them guessing what the secret low GI ingredient is – and we're not talking about the cloudy apple juice. Don't spill the beans before you enjoy the compliments. PS: This cake should be frozen after 1 day, as the lentil taste becomes stronger with time.

Makes 10 slices **Preparation time** 25 minutes
Cooking time 50 minutes + cooling time

½ cup (125 g) red lentils, picked over and rinsed
1½ cups (375 ml) unsweetened cloudy apple juice
¾ cup (110 g) gluten-free self-raising flour
⅓ cup (40 g) cocoa
⅔ cup (80 g) almond meal
4 eggs, separated
⅔ cup (150 g) caster sugar
½ teaspoon almond essence
pure icing sugar or gluten-free icing sugar mixture (optional)

To serve
low fat vanilla ice-cream

1 Preheat the oven to 180°C. Grease and line a 20 cm-base round cake pan.

2 Place the lentils and apple juice in a small saucepan. Bring to the boil, reduce the heat and simmer, stirring occasionally, for 15 minutes or until lentils are soft. Set aside to cool.

3 Sift the flour and cocoa into a bowl, stir to combine, then sift a second time to aerate. Stir in the almond meal.

4 Beat the egg yolks and sugar in a large bowl until pale and creamy. Fold in the cooled lentil mix, sifted flour and almond essence and stir to combine.

5 Place the egg whites in a bowl and beat until firm peaks form. Fold into the chocolate cake mix.

6 Pour the batter into the prepared cake pan. Bake for 30–35 minutes or until the top is firm and a skewer inserted into the centre comes out clean. Remove from the oven and leave in pan for 5 minutes before turning out onto a wire rack to cool. Dust the top with icing sugar before serving with ice-cream if you wish.

PER SLICE WITHOUT ICE-CREAM
966 kJ; 7 g fat (including 1.5 g saturated fat); 2.5 g fibre; 7 g protein; 34 g carbohydrate

Cranberry Baked Apples

Stuffed baked apples are easy to prepare and a great way to boost your fruit intake. Try them with our other filling options at the end of the recipe.

Serves 4 **Preparation time** 15 minutes **Cooking time** 40–45 minutes

⅓ cup (40 g) finely chopped walnuts
⅓ cup (55 g) craisins (dried cranberries)
2 tablespoons pure maple syrup
1 teaspoon cinnamon
4 medium-sized green apples
1 cup (250 ml) unsweetened cloudy apple juice

To serve

low fat vanilla ice-cream or low fat plain yoghurt blended with cinnamon and runny honey or maple syrup, to taste

1. Preheat the oven to 180°C.

2. To make the walnut stuffing, combine the walnuts, craisins, maple syrup and cinnamon in a bowl.

3. Core the apples and run a knife lightly around the centre of the apple (horizontally) to make a shallow cut. Stuff the apples with an equal amount of the walnut mixture and arrange them in an ovenproof dish that fits the four apples snugly. Any leftover filling can be placed in the dish. Pour the apple juice over the apples and cover the dish with a lid or foil.

4. Bake for 40–45 minutes, or until the apples are tender when tested with a skewer, basting apples with cooking juices halfway through. To serve, place an apple on each serving plate and drizzle a little of the pan juices over. Serve with ice-cream or yoghurt if desired.

VARIATIONS

- For a stuffing that the kids will love, mix ⅓ cup (50 g) chopped dried apricots with ¼ cup (45 g) white choc bits and 1 tablespoon apple juice.
- Mix ⅔ cup (130 g) sultanas with 1 teaspoon cinnamon, 2 teaspoons brown sugar, ½ teaspoon vanilla essence and 1 tablespoon apple juice – and use as the filling instead.
- Mix ¼ cup (35 g) chopped dried apricots, ¼ cup (40 g) craisins, ¼ cup (35 g) chopped macadamia nuts, 2 teaspoons brown sugar and 1 tablespoon apple juice – and use as the filling instead.

PER SERVE WITHOUT ICE-CREAM OR YOGHURT TOPPING
1056 kJ; 8 g fat (including 0.5 g saturated fat); 4.5 g fibre; 2 g protein; 43 g carbohydrate

Lemon Delicious Pudding

Lemon Delicious Pudding really is delicious. The name says it all. For a special occasion when you want to end the meal with a tangy taste, this is the pudding to serve.

Serves 6 **Preparation time** 20 minutes **Cooking time** 35 minutes

¼ cup (35 g) rice flour
¼ teaspoon gluten-free baking powder
2 teaspoons rice bran
60 g reduced-fat margarine
½ cup (110 g) caster sugar
1 tablespoon grated lemon rind
3 eggs, separated
2 tablespoons lemon juice
1 cup (250 ml) reduced-fat milk

1. Preheat the oven to 180°C. Grease a 1½-litre-capacity soufflé or ovenproof baking dish.

2. Sift the flour, baking powder and bran into a bowl, stir and then sift again to aerate.

3. Cream the margarine, sugar and lemon rind in a mixing bowl until light and creamy. Add the egg yolks, one at a time, beating well after each addition. Fold in the sifted flour mixture and then stir in the lemon juice and milk, mixing until smooth.

4. Beat the egg whites in a medium bowl until firm peaks form. Fold lightly into the lemon mixture.

5. Pour the mixture into the prepared baking dish. Place the baking dish in a larger pan filled with boiling water to reach halfway up the side of the pudding dish. Bake for 35 minutes or until the top is golden.

PER SERVE
806 kJ; 8 g fat (including 2 g saturated fat); negligible fibre; 5.5 g protein; 25 g carbohydrate

Rhubarb and Apple Crumble

Everyone loves a crumble on a wintry night. It's the ultimate comfort dessert. We've added fibre to this one with rice bran cereal – it can be crushed lightly in a food processor. There's no need to process it to a powder, just chop up the sticks.

2 green apples, peeled, quartered, cored and thinly sliced
3 tablespoons caster sugar
¼ cup (60 ml) orange juice
1 bunch rhubarb, trimmed and cut into about 5 cm pieces
1 teaspoon grated orange rind

Crumble
1 tablespoon rice flour
1 tablespoon gluten-free cornflour
⅓ cup (40 g) almond meal
½ cup (60 g) lightly crushed rice bran cereal
¼ cup (50 g) brown sugar
½ teaspoon cinnamon
¼ teaspoon ground ginger
25 g reduced-fat margarine
¼ cup (30 g) slivered almonds

To serve
low fat vanilla ice-cream or yoghurt

1. Preheat the oven to 200°C. Grease a 1½-litre ovenproof dish.

2. Place the apples, sugar and juice in a medium-sized saucepan. Bring just to the boil, then reduce the heat to low, cover, and cook for 10 minutes. Add the rhubarb, cover, and cook for another 10 minutes. Remove from the heat, stir in the orange rind, and set aside to cool for 10 minutes. Spoon into the prepared dish (use a slotted spoon if there is too much liquid).

3. To make the crumble, combine the rice flour, cornflour, almond meal, rice bran cereal, sugar, cinnamon and ginger. Rub in the margarine until combined. Stir in the slivered almonds. Spoon the crumble evenly over the fruit. Bake for 20 minutes or until the top is brown and crunchy. Serve with ice-cream or yoghurt if desired.

VARIATION
- If you are short of time you could use your favourite gluten-free muesli to make the topping.

PER SERVE WITHOUT ICE-CREAM OR YOGHURT
1490 kJ; 14 g fat (including 1.5 g saturated fat); 6.5 g fibre; 6 g protein; 49 g carbohydrate

Orange Almond Dessert Cake

This is a deliciously moist, dense and rich dessert cake inspired by Claudia Roden's famous Middle Eastern orange and almond cake. It is very easy to make, but you do need to set aside the time to cook the oranges. It doesn't need an accompaniment, as it is very rich. This will keep for about 5 days in the refrigerator, but is unsuitable for freezing.

Makes 16 slices **Preparation time** 25 minutes
Cooking time 2 hours 45 minutes + cooling time

2 large (about 250 g each) oranges, washed
400 g can chickpeas, drained and rinsed
5 eggs, separated
1¼ cups (280 g) caster sugar
125 g ground almonds
1 teaspoon gluten-free baking powder
1 teaspoon vanilla essence

1 Place the oranges (skin and all) in a saucepan with a little water (enough to cover ⅓–½ of the oranges). Bring to the boil, cover and cook, turning occasionally, for 1¼–1½ hours or until oranges are soft. Remove oranges from the liquid and leave to cool. When cool, quarter, remove the white stalk and pips, and chop roughly.

2 Meanwhile, preheat the oven to 170°C. Grease and line the base of a 25 cm-base round cake pan.

3 Place chickpeas in a food processor and process until chopped. Add the oranges and process again until puréed.

4 Beat the egg yolks and sugar together in a very large bowl until thick, pale and creamy. Fold in the orange purée, almonds, baking powder and vanilla essence until combined.

5 Whisk the egg whites in a bowl until soft peaks form. Fold into the orange mixture.

6 Pour the cake batter into the cake pan. Bake for 1 hour and 15 minutes or until top is firm, cake is not wobbly and a skewer inserted into the centre comes out almost clean. If the top of the cake is turning too brown after the first 50 minutes, you may need to cover the cake with foil.

7 Remove the cake from the oven and allow to rest in the pan for 20 minutes. Turn out onto a wire rack, then turn the right way up to cool completely.

PER SLICE
692 kJ; 6 g fat (including 1 g saturated fat); 2 g fibre; 5 g protein; 23 g carbohydrate

Tips for using legumes in your baking

- Canned legumes such as chickpeas are suitable for baking, but only for dense, robust cakes. Wash and drain beans well then purée. Experiment with different types.
- Use strong flavours such as vanilla essence, coconut essence, almond essence, cocoa, or lots of lemon, orange or lime zest to mask the savoury taste of the legumes. You might need to increase the amount of sugar in the cake by a small amount.
- Chickpeas add a nutty flavour and a pleasant, coarse texture. They go well with lemons and oranges.
- If flour is used in the recipe, use a commercial gluten-free flour as these usually produce a better result with legumes than combining different types of gluten-free flours.

Yoghurt Strawberry Jelly

Definitely one for the children!

Serves 4 **Preparation time** 10 minutes + setting time

85 g packet strawberry-flavoured jelly crystals
1 punnet (200 g) chopped strawberries
1½ cups (300 g) low fat strawberry yoghurt

To serve

low fat ice-cream
chopped, toasted nuts

1 Combine the jelly crystals and 1 cup (250 ml) boiling water in a bowl, and stir until dissolved. Place in the refrigerator to cool – but do not allow to set. (It is quicker to cool it in the freezer, but watch that it doesn't set.)

2 When cool, fold the strawberries and yoghurt through the jelly and mix well. Spoon evenly into tall serving glasses, cover and refrigerate until set. Serve topped with a scoop of low fat ice-cream and a sprinkle of your favourite toasted nuts.

VARIATION
- Replace the strawberry yoghurt with low fat vanilla yoghurt.

PER SERVE WITH ICE-CREAM AND NUTS
905 kJ; 4 g fat (including 1 g saturated fat); 1.5 g fibre; 8 g protein; 36 g carbohydrate

Chapter 13: Basics

Stocks, sauces, dips, mashes and spice blends to add that final flourish to a meal or snack.

How to poach chicken and end up with a delicious chicken stock, too

Chicken poached in an aromatic stock is ideal for salads, and the meat turns out so juicy and tender. Strain the stock and use it when making soups and stews.

Preparation time 10 minutes **Cooking time** 15 minutes + cooling time

2 skinless chicken breast fillets
1 carrot, chopped into chunks
1 stick celery, sliced
2–3 stems coriander or parsley, roughly chopped
1 bay leaf
1 clove garlic, crushed (optional)
2.5 cm piece fresh ginger, chopped
1 tablespoon black peppercorns

1 Place the chicken breast fillets in a saucepan with the remaining ingredients. Cover with cold water. Bring to the boil, then reduce the heat to low and simmer for 10 minutes. Set aside to cool in the poaching liquid for an hour. When cool enough to handle, use a fork to shred the chicken or cut into bite-sized pieces.

Hommous

Makes about 1½ cups **Preparation time** 5 minutes

1⅓ cups (225 g) cooked or canned chickpeas
¼ cup (70 g) tahini
2 cloves garlic, peeled
3 tablespoons lemon juice
2 tablespoons olive oil
salt (optional)
freshly ground black pepper

1 Place the chickpeas, tahini, garlic, lemon juice and oil in a small food processor. Process until well combined and smooth. Add 2–3 tablespoons hot water to thin the mixture slightly. Season to taste with salt and pepper. Store in an airtight container in the refrigerator for up to 2 weeks.

Easy Guacamole

Makes about 1 cup **Preparation time** 2 minutes

1 avocado
1 tablespoon lemon juice
1 tablespoon snipped chives, parsley or coriander

1. In a small bowl, mash the avocado and lemon juice with a fork and mix in the chives, parsley or coriander.

Potato and Cannellini Mash

Serves 4 **Preparation time** 10 minutes **Cooking time** 25 minutes

about 400 g Carisma, Nicola or small chat potatoes
2 cloves garlic, peeled
400 g can cannellini beans, drained and rinsed
2 teaspoons reduced-fat margarine
¼ cup (60 ml) hot skim milk
2 tablespoons chopped chives
freshly ground black pepper

1. Place the potatoes and garlic cloves in a medium-sized saucepan and cover with cold water. Bring to the boil and cook for about 15 minutes or until potatoes are tender. Drain. When cool enough, peel the potatoes.

2. Mash the potatoes, garlic and beans with a potato masher.

3. Melt the margarine in a saucepan. Add the mashed mixture with milk and stir for 1–2 minutes until warm. Stir in the chives and season with pepper.

Lentil Mash

Serves 4 **Preparation time** 5 minutes **Cooking time** 25 minutes

1 cup (250 g) red lentils, picked over and rinsed
2½ cups (625 ml) gluten-free reduced-salt chicken stock
1 tablespoon fresh thyme leaves
freshly ground black pepper

1. Place the lentils, stock and thyme in a medium saucepan. Bring to the boil. Reduce heat and simmer for 20 minutes, stirring occasionally towards the end to prevent lentils from sticking to pan base, or until the lentils are soft and the liquid has evaporated. Season to taste.

Sweet Potato Mash

Serves 4 **Preparation time** 10 minutes **Cooking time** 15 minutes

400 g orange sweet potato, peeled and cubed
400 g can cannellini beans, drained and rinsed
2 teaspoons reduced-fat margarine
freshly ground black pepper
1 tablespoon chopped basil (optional)
2 teaspoons balsamic vinegar (optional)

1. Boil, steam or microwave the sweet potato until tender. Place the sweet potato and beans in a food processor and process until roughly mashed. Transfer to a bowl.

2. To reheat the sweet potatoes, melt the margarine in a medium-sized saucepan, then add the mash. Stir over low heat for about 2–3 minutes or until heated through. Season with pepper, add basil and vinegar, if using, and stir through the mash.

Chipotle Chilli in Adobo Sauce

Makes 1 cup **Preparation time** 5 minutes **Cooking time** 1–1½ hours

7 medium-sized dried chipotle chillies, stems removed
⅓ cup sliced onion
5 tablespoons (100 ml) cider vinegar
2 cloves garlic, chopped
¼ cup (60 ml) tomato sauce
¼ teaspoon salt
3 cups (750 ml) water

1. Combine all the ingredients in a medium-sized saucepan. Cover and cook over a low heat for 1–1½ hours or until the chillies are very soft and the liquid has been reduced to 1 cup. This recipe will keep for 2–3 weeks in an airtight container in the refrigerator.

Italian Herb Blend

1 tablespoon dried basil
3 teaspoons dried thyme
2 teaspoons dried marjoram
2 teaspoons dried oregano

1 teaspoon dried sage
1 teaspoon dried garlic flakes
1 teaspoon dried rosemary

Madras Curry Blend

4 tablespoons ground coriander seed
1¼ tablespoons (5 teaspoons) ground cumin
3 teaspoons ground turmeric
2 teaspoons ground ginger
1 teaspoon ground yellow mustard seed
1 teaspoon ground fenugreek seed

1 teaspoon ground cinnamon
½ teaspoon ground cloves
½ teaspoon ground cardamom seed
½ teaspoon (or more to taste) ground chilli
1½ teaspoons freshly ground black pepper

Gluten-free spice blends

You may have already discovered that many spice blends in your supermarket contain gluten in the form of wheat starch. That's why we recommend Herbie's brand for our recipes – apart from asafoetida (which contains wheat starch) and blends that contain asafoetida, Herbie's blends and spices are gluten-free. See page 248 for contact details.

Strawberry Sauce

This is a much better version of the strawberry sauce that you get from the supermarket. And, of course, it tastes like real strawberries! It's so easy to make. Double the quantities when strawberries are in season (and more affordable). Pour over ice-cream, mix through plain yoghurt, serve with fruit, or use in place of chocolate sauce on a banana split.

Makes 1 cup **Preparation time** 5 minutes

200 g (1 punnet) strawberries, washed, hulled and chopped
2 teaspoons caster sugar

1. Place strawberries and sugar in a food processor and process until smooth. Keep refrigerated.

The GI gluten-free tables

Using the tables

These tables will help you put low GI food choices into your shopping trolley and onto your plate. Each entry lists an individual food and its GI value. We also list a nominal serve size, the amount of carbohydrate per serve, the GL and whether the food's GI is low, medium or high.

While the tables list only gluten-free foods, on page 213 we have included information about wheat-free but not gluten-free cereals.

> A low GI value is 55 or less
> A medium/moderate GI value is 56 to 69 inclusive
> A high GI value is 70 or more

You can use the tables to:

- Find the GI of your favourite foods
- Compare carb-rich foods within a category (two types of bread or breakfast cereal, for example)
- Identify the best carbohydrate choices
- Improve your diet by finding a low GI substitute for high GI foods
- Put together a low GI meal, and
- Find foods with a high GI but low GL

Each individual food appears alphabetically within a food category, such as 'Bread' or 'Fruit'. This makes it easy to compare the kinds of foods you eat every day and helps you see which high GI foods you could substitute with low GI versions.

The food categories used in the tables are:

- Beans, peas and legumes – including baked beans, chickpeas, lentils and split peas
- Beverages – including fruit and vegetable juices, soft drinks, flavoured milk and sport drinks
- Biscuits – including commercial sweet biscuits, savoury crispbreads and plain crackers
- Bread – including sliced white and wholemeal bread, fruit breads and flatbreads
- Breakfast cereals – including processed cereals, muesli, oats and porridge
- Wheat-free breakfast cereals
- Cakes and muffins – including other baked goods
- Cereal grains

- Dairy products – including milk, yoghurt, ice-creams and dairy desserts
- Fast food and convenience meals
- Fruit – including fresh, canned and dried fruit
- Gluten-free products
- Meat, seafood and protein
- Pasta and noodles
- Rice
- Snack foods – including chocolate, fruit bars, muesli bars and nuts
- Soy products – including soy milk and soy yoghurt
- Spreads and sweeteners – including sugars, honey and jam
- Vegetables – including green vegetables, salad vegetables and root vegetables

In the tables you will sometimes see these symbols:

★ indicates that a food contains little or no carbohydrate. We have included these foods – including vegetables and protein-rich foods – because so many people ask us for their GI.

■ indicates that a food is high in saturated fat. Not all low GI foods are a good choice; some are too high in saturated fat and sodium for everyday eating. Remember to consider the overall nutritional value of a food.

Ⓖ indicates that a food is part of the GI symbol program. Foods with the GI symbol have had their GI tested properly and are a healthy choice for their food category.

To make a fair comparison, all foods have been tested using an internationally standardised method. Gram for gram of carbohydrates, the higher the GI, the higher the blood glucose levels after consumption. If you can't find the GI value for a food you regularly eat in these tables, check out our website (www.glycemicindex.com). We maintain an international database of published GI values that have been tested by a reliable laboratory. Alternatively, please write to the manufacturer and encourage them to have the food tested by an accredited laboratory such as Sydney University's Glycemic Index Research Service (SUGiRS). In the meantime, choose a similar food from the tables as a substitute.

The GI values in this book are correct at the time of publication. However, the formulation of commercial foods can change and the GI can change, too. You can rely on foods showing the GI symbol. Although some manufacturers include the GI on the nutritional label, you would need to know that the testing was carried out independently by an accredited laboratory.

FOOD	NOMINAL SERVE SIZE g/ml	CARB (g)	GI	LOW MED HIGH
BEANS, PEAS & LEGUMES				
Baked beans, canned in tomato sauce	150	17	49	low
Baked beans, canned in tomato sauce, Heinz®	150	17	55	low
Beans, canned refried, Casa Fiesta	113	20	38	low
Black beans, boiled	150	25	30	low
Black-eyed beans, soaked, boiled	150	29	42	low
Borlotti beans, canned, drained, Edgell	75	12	41	low
Broad beans	80	11	79	high
Butter beans, canned, drained, Edgell	75	12	36	low
Butter beans, dried, boiled	150	20	31	low
Butter beans, soaked overnight, boiled 50 mins	150	75	26	low
Cannellini beans	85	12	31	low
Chickpeas, canned in brine	150	22	40	low
Chickpeas, dried, boiled	150	24	28	low
Four bean mix, canned, drained, Edgell	75	12	37	low
Haricot beans, cooked, canned	150	31	38	low
Haricot beans, dried, boiled	150	31	33	low
Kidney beans, dark red, canned, drained	150	25	43	low
Kidney beans, red, canned, drained, Edgell	150	17	36	low
Kidney beans, red, dried, boiled	150	25	28	low

★ little or no carbs   ■ high in saturated fat   ⓒ GI Symbol partner

FOOD	NOMINAL SERVE SIZE g/ml	CARB (g)	GI	LOW MED HIGH
BEANS, PEAS & LEGUMES (CONT.)				
Kidney beans, red, soaked overnight, boiled 60 mins	150	60	51	low
Lentils, green, canned	150	17	48	low
Lentils, green, dried, boiled	150	17	30	low
Lentils, red, dried, boiled	150	18	26	low
Lentils, red, split, boiled 25 mins	150	77	21	low
Lima beans, baby, frozen, reheated	150	30	32	low
Mung beans	150	17	39	low
Peas, dried, boiled	150	9	22	low
Peas, green, frozen, boiled	80	7	48	low
Snake beans	70	0	★	
Soy beans, canned, drained	150	6	14	low
Soy beans, dried, boiled	150	6	18	low
Split peas, yellow, boiled 20 mins	150	19	32	low
Split peas, yellow, dried, soaked overnight, boiled 55 mins	150	32	25	low

★ little or no carbs ■ high in saturated fat ⓒ GI Symbol partner

FOOD	NOMINAL SERVE SIZE g/ml	CARB (g)	GI	LOW MED HIGH
BEVERAGES				
Apple and Blackcurrant juice, pure, Berri	250	26	43	low
ⓖ Apple and Cherry juice, pure, Wild About Fruit®	250	33	43	low
ⓖ Apple and Mango juice, pure, Wild About Fruit®	250	34	47	low
ⓖ Apple juice, filtered, pure, Wild About Fruit®	250	30	44	low
Apple juice, Granny Smith, unsweetened, Ducat's	250	30	44	low
Apple juice, no added sugar	250	28	40	low
ⓖ Apple juice with fibre, Wild About Fruit®	250	28	37	low
ⓖ Apple, pineapple and passionfruit juice, Wild About Fruit®	250	33	48	low
Big M Chocolate flavoured milk	250	24	37	low
Big M Strawberry flavoured milk	250	24	37	low
Build-Up, drink powder, vanilla with fibre, in water, Nestlé®	250	35	41	low
Carrot juice, freshly made	250	23	43	low
Coca-Cola®	250	26	53	low
Coffee, black, no milk or sugar	250	0	★	
Cordial, orange, reconstituted	250	20	66	med
Cranberry Juice Cocktail, Ocean Spray	250	31	52	low
Diet soft drink	250	0	★	

★ little or no carbs   ■ high in saturated fat   ⓖ GI Symbol partner

FOOD	NOMINAL SERVE SIZE g/ml	CARB (g)	GI	LOW MED HIGH
BEVERAGES (CONT.)				
Ensure™, vanilla drink	250	34	48	low
Fanta®, orange soft drink	250	34	68	med
Gatorade®	250	15	78	high
Grapefruit juice, unsweetened	250	22	48	low
Isostar®	250	18	70	high
Jevity®, fibre-enriched drink	237	36	48	low
Lucozade®, original, sparkling glucose drink	250	42	95	high
Mango smoothie	250	27	32	low
Nesquik® powder, Chocolate, in 1.5% fat milk	250	11	41	low
Orange juice, unsweetened, fresh	250	18	50	low
Orange juice, unsweetened, from concentrate, Quelch	250	18	53	low
Pineapple juice, unsweetened	250	34	46	low
Prune juice, Golden Circle Healthy Life Natural	200	30	43	low
Ribena Blackcurrant fruit syrup (reconstituted)	250	32	52	low
Schweppes Lemonade	250	28	54	low
Solo®, lemon squash soft drink	250	29	58	med
Sustagen® Drink, Dutch Chocolate	250	41	31	low

★ little or no carbs ■ high in saturated fat ⓒ GI Symbol partner

FOOD	NOMINAL SERVE SIZE g/ml	CARB (g)	GI	LOW MED HIGH
BEVERAGES (CONT.)				
Sustagen Sport®, milk-based drink	250	49	43	low
ⓖ Thorpedo advanced hydration for kids, Berry Blaster	350	49	16	low
ⓖ Thorpedo advanced hydration for kids, Troppo	350	49	11	low
ⓖ Thorpedo Ultra Low GI Energy Water, Berry	600	27	16	low
ⓖ Thorpedo Ultra Low GI Energy Water, Lemon Lime	600	27	16	low
ⓖ Thorpedo Ultra Low GI Energy Water, Orange	600	27	19	low
ⓖ Thorpedo Ultra Low GI Energy Water, Tropical	600	27	16	low
Tomato juice, no added sugar, Berri	250	9	38	low

★ little or no carbs   ■ high in saturated fat   ⓖ GI Symbol partner

FOOD	NOMINAL SERVE SIZE g/ml	CARB (g)	GI	LOW MED HIGH
BISCUITS				
Corn Thins, Real Foods, puffed corn cakes, gluten-free	25	20	87	high
Puffed Rice Cakes, white, Ricegrowers	25	21	82	high

★ little or no carbs ■ high in saturated fat © GI Symbol partner

FOOD	NOMINAL SERVE SIZE g/ml	CARB (g)	GI	LOW MED HIGH
BREAD				
Buckwheat bread (Gluten and Wheat Free), Naturis Bakery	30	11	72	high
Country Life Low GI Gluten Free white	30	8	53	low
Country Life multi-grain bread	30	13	79	high
Diego's White Corn Tortillas	56	28	53	low
Woolworth's Select White Corn Tortillas	50	24	53	low

★ little or no carbs   ■ high in saturated fat   Ⓖ GI Symbol partner

FOOD	NOMINAL SERVE SIZE g/ml	CARB (g)	GI	LOW MED HIGH
BREAKFAST CEREALS				
Muesli, gluten and wheat free with psyllium, Freedom Foods	40	13	50	low
Puffed buckwheat	14	12	65	med
Rice Bran, extruded, Ricegrowers	30	14	19	low

★ little or no carbs ■ high in saturated fat ☺ GI Symbol partner

FOOD	NOMINAL SERVE SIZE g/ml	CARB (g)	GI	LOW MED HIGH
WHEAT-FREE BREAKFAST CEREALS (NOT GLUTEN-FREE)				
Digestive 1st, Goodness Superfoods	45	21	39	low
Fibreboost Sprinkles 1st, Goodness Superfoods	15	6	34	low
Heart 1st, Goodness Superfoods	45	20	46	low
Oat bran, raw, unprocessed	10	5	55	low
Oats, rolled, raw, Lowan®	50	31	59	med
Porridge, instant, made with water, Uncle Tobys	30	26	82	high
Porridge, made from steel-cut oats with water	40	22	52	low
Porridge, multigrain, made with water, Monster Muesli	60	21	55	low
Porridge, regular, made from oats with water	250	21	58	med
Protein 1st, Goodness Superfoods	45	17	36	low
Quick Barley + Oats 1st, Goodness Superfoods	35	16	53	low
Quick Barley + Oats 1st Apple + Honey, Goodness Superfoods	35	21	55	low
Quick Oats Porridge, Freedom Foods	30	19	50	low
Traditional Barley + Oats 1st, Goodness Superfoods	40	18	47	low

★ little or no carbs ■ high in saturated fat ☉ GI Symbol partner

FOOD	NOMINAL SERVE SIZE g/ml	CARB (g)	GI	LOW MED HIGH
CAKES & MUFFINS				
Pancakes, buckwheat, gluten-free, packet mix, Orgran	77	22	102	high

★ little or no carbs ■ high in saturated fat ⊙ GI Symbol partner

FOOD	NOMINAL SERVE SIZE g/ml	CARB (g)	GI	LOW MED HIGH
CEREAL GRAINS				
Buckwheat, boiled	150	30	54	low
Millet, boiled	150	36	71	high
Polenta (cornmeal), boiled	150	13	68	med
Quinoa, boiled	100	17	51	low

★ little or no carbs   ■ high in saturated fat   ☺ GI Symbol partner

FOOD	NOMINAL SERVE SIZE g/ml	CARB (g)	GI	LOW MED HIGH
DAIRY PRODUCTS—ICE-CREAM, CUSTARDS & DESSERTS				
Cheese	40	0	★■	
Chocolate Mousse, Diet, Nestlé®	50	11	31	low
Crème Caramel, Diet, Nestlé®	125	12	33	low
Custard, Trim, vanilla, reduced-fat, Paul's®	100	15	37	low
Fruche Apricot Vanilla and Honey	150	22	34	low
Fruche Lemon Meringue	150	19	41	low
Fruche Vanilla Crème	150	22	49	low
Frutia™, low fat frozen fruit dessert, Mango, Weiss	100	23	42	low
Gelati, Alba, sucrose-free, chocolate	50	14	37	low
Gelati, Alba, sucrose-free, vanilla	50	14	39	low
Health Plus Dairy Snack, Paul's®, Lemon Cream	165	33	32	low
Health Plus Dairy Snack, Paul's®, Raspberry Cream	165	33	32	low
Health Plus Dairy Snack, Paul's®, Vanilla Cream	165	34	35	low
Ⓖ Ice-cream, Bulla Light creamy low fat, chocolate	65	17	27	low
Ⓖ Ice-cream, Bulla Light creamy low fat, English toffee	65	17	27	low

★ little or no carbs ■ high in saturated fat Ⓖ GI Symbol partner

DAIRY PRODUCTS—ICE-CREAM, CUSTARDS & DESSERTS (CONT.)

FOOD	NOMINAL SERVE SIZE g/ml	CARB (g)	GI	LOW MED HIGH
ⓖ Ice-cream, Bulla Light creamy low fat, mango	65	17	30	low
ⓖ Ice-cream, Bulla Light creamy low fat, vanilla	65	13	36	low
Ice-cream, Sara Lee®, full fat, French Vanilla	50	9	38 ■	low
Ice-cream, Sara Lee®, full fat, Ultra Chocolate	50	9	37 ■	low
Nestlé® Diet Lemon Cheesecake	120	12	31	low
Tapioca pudding, boiled, with milk	250	18	81	high
Vanilla pudding, Sustagen®, instant, made from powdered mix	250	47	27	low
Yoplait Le Rice, dairy rice desserts, Apple Cinnamon	180	38	52	low
Yoplait Le Rice, dairy rice desserts, Caramel	180	38	41	low
Yoplait Le Rice, dairy rice desserts, Classic Vanilla	180	33	36	low
Yoplait Le Rice, dairy rice desserts, Forest Berries	180	36	45	low
Yoplait Le Rice, dairy rice desserts, Raspberry and Apple	180	38	52	low
Yoplait Le Rice, dairy rice desserts, Strawberry	180	38	54	low

★ little or no carbs   ■ high in saturated fat   ⓖ GI Symbol partner

FOOD	NOMINAL SERVE SIZE g/ml	CARB (g)	GI	LOW MED HIGH
DAIRY PRODUCTS—ICE-CREAM, CUSTARDS & DESSERTS (CONT.)				
Yoplait Le Rice, dairy rice desserts, Tropical Mango	180	38	54	low
Yoplait Le Rice, dairy rice desserts, Vanilla	180	37	43	low

★ little or no carbs   ■ high in saturated fat   © GI Symbol partner

FOOD	NOMINAL SERVE SIZE g/ml	CARB (g)	GI	LOW MED HIGH
DAIRY PRODUCTS—MILK & ALTERNATIVES				
Australia's Own natural rice low fat drink	250	34	92	high
Big M Chocolate flavoured milk	250	24	37	low
Big M Strawberry flavoured milk	250	24	37	low
Condensed milk, sweetened, full fat	50	28	61 ■	med
ⓖ Lite White, reduced-fat (1.4%) milk, Dairy Farmers™	250	14	30	low
Milk (3.6% fat)	250	12	27 ■	low
Pura HiLo Milk	250	14	20	low
Pura Light Start milk	250	15	30	low
Pura Skimmer Milk	250	14	20	low
Pura Tone Milk	250	16	30	low
Rush™ Intense Coffee, Paul's®	250	14	24	low
Rush™, low fat flavoured milk, Absolute Caramel, Paul's®	100	11	42	low
Rush™, low fat flavoured milk, Ultimate Chocolate, Paul's®	100	10	38	low
Rush™, low fat flavoured milk, Wicked Latte, Paul's®	100	10	38	low
Rush™, low fat flavoured milk, Wild Strawberry, Paul's®	100	10	38	low
Shape, calcium-enriched, low fat (0.1%) milk	250	17	34	low
ⓖ Skim, low fat (0.1%) milk, Dairy Farmers™	250	12	32	low

★ little or no carbs   ■ high in saturated fat   ⓖ GI Symbol partner

FOOD	NOMINAL SERVE SIZE g/ml	CARB (g)	GI	LOW MED HIGH
DAIRY PRODUCTS—MILK & ALTERNATIVES (CONT.)				
ⓖ Take Care, calcium-enriched, reduced fat (1%) milk, Dairy Farmers™	250	15	23	low
Vitasoy®, rice milk, calcium-enriched	250	22	79	high
Vitasoy ®, chocolate, reduced fat, soy milk	250	19	31	low
Vitasoy ®, vanilla, reduced fat, soy milk	250	17	31	low
Vitasoy ® So Milky, regular, soy milk	250	8	21	low
Vitasoy ® So Milky, lite, soy milk	250	7	17	low

★ little or no carbs ■ high in saturated fat ⓖ GI Symbol partner

FOOD	NOMINAL SERVE SIZE g/ml	CARB (g)	GI	LOW MED HIGH
DAIRY PRODUCTS—YOGHURT				
ⓖ Brownes Diet No Fat Yoghurt Apricot Danish	200	16	24	low
ⓖ Brownes Diet No Fat Yoghurt Black Cherry	200	15	24	low
ⓖ Brownes Diet No Fat Yoghurt Sticky Date Pudding	200	17	40	low
ⓖ Brownes Diet No Fat Yoghurt Strawberry Sundae	200	15	40	low
Diet, low fat, no added sugar, vanilla or fruit	200	13	20	low
Jalna Bio Dynamic, Bush Honey	200	13	26	low
Jalna Fat Free, Natural	200	7	19	low
Jalna Fat Free, Passionfruit	200	14	27	low
Jalna Leben European-style	200	7	11	low
Jalna Premium Blend, Creamy Vanilla	200	15	18	low
Jalna Premium Blend, Greek-style	200	8	12	low
Jalna Yoghurt on the Go, Wildberry	200	13	19	low
ⓖ Nestlé® All Natural 99% Fat Free Plain Natural	200	16	14	low
ⓖ Nestlé® All Natural Light Apricot	200	31	49	low
ⓖ Nestlé® All Natural Light Banana	200	22	38	low
ⓖ Nestlé® All Natural Light Forest Berry	200	30	37	low
ⓖ Nestlé® All Natural Light Mango	200	33	55	low

★ little or no carbs　■ high in saturated fat　ⓖ GI Symbol partner

FOOD	NOMINAL SERVE SIZE g/ml	CARB (g)	GI	LOW MED HIGH
DAIRY PRODUCTS—YOGHURT (CONT.)				
⒢ Nestlé® All Natural Light Passionfruit	200	30	47	low
⒢ Nestlé® All Natural Light Strawberry	200	31	37	low
⒢ Nestlé® All Natural Light Tropical Fruit Salad	200	22	38	low
⒢ Nestlé® All Natural Light Vanilla	200	31	37	low
⒢ Nestlé® diet, low fat, all flavours	200	11	19–21	low
Ski d'Lite™, low fat, with sugar, Honey Buzz	200	36	47	low
Ski d'Lite™, low fat, with sugar, Vanilla Crème	200	32	46	low
Ski d'Lite™, low fat, with sugar, Wild Strawberry	200	30	31	low
Vaalia®, low fat with sugar, Apricot, Mango and Peach	100	15	26	low
Vaalia®, low fat with sugar, French Vanilla	100	18	26	low
Vaalia®, low fat with sugar, Lemon Crème	100	19	43	low
Vaalia®, low fat with sugar, Luscious Berries	100	15	28	low
Vaalia®, low fat with sugar, Passionfruit	100	17	32	low
Vaalia®, low fat with sugar, Tempting Strawberry	100	15	28	low
Vaalia®, no fat with sugar, French Vanilla	150	27	40	low
Vaalia®, no fat with sugar, Mango	150	25	39	low
Vaalia®, no fat with sugar, Tempting Strawberry	150	22	38	low

★ little or no carbs ■ high in saturated fat ⒢ GI Symbol partner

FOOD	NOMINAL SERVE SIZE g/ml	CARB (g)	GI	LOW MED HIGH
DAIRY PRODUCTS—YOGHURT (CONT.)				
Vaalia®, no fat with sugar, Wild Berries	150	22	38	low
Yakult™, fermented probiotic milk drink	65	12	46	low
Yakult™ Light, fermented probiotic milk drink	65	9	36	low
Yoplait Lite Apple Tart yoghurt	200	32	27	low
Yoplait Lite Apricot yoghurt	200	31	27	low
Yoplait Lite Berry Bliss yoghurt	200	32	25	low
Yoplait Lite Blueberry Crème yoghurt	200	34	25	low
Yoplait Lite Blueberry yoghurt	200	34	25	low
Yoplait Lite Creamy Vanilla yoghurt	200	35	27	low
Yoplait Lite Field Strawberries yoghurt	200	34	25	low
Yoplait Lite French Cheesecake yoghurt	200	37	27	low
Yoplait Lite Fruit Salad yoghurt	200	27	32	low
Yoplait Lite Lemon Meringue yoghurt	200	32	27	low
Yoplait Lite Mango Passion yoghurt	200	32	37	low
Yoplait Lite Mango yoghurt	200	33	37	low
Yoplait Lite Passionfruit yoghurt	200	31	37	low
Yoplait Lite Peach Mango yoghurt	200	31	37	low
Yoplait Lite Rhubarb Custard yoghurt	200	33	27	low
Yoplait Lite Strawberry yoghurt	200	32	25	low
Yoplait Lite Tropical Mango yoghurt	200	27	32	low

★ little or no carbs   ■ high in saturated fat   ⓒ GI Symbol partner

DAIRY PRODUCTS—YOGHURT (CONT.)

FOOD	NOMINAL SERVE SIZE g/ml	CARB (g)	GI	LOW MED HIGH
Yoplait Lite Tropical yoghurt	200	32	37	low
Yoplait Lite Vanilla Strawberry yoghurt	200	34	25	low
Yoplait No Fat Apple Pie yoghurt	200	14	18	low
Yoplait No Fat Apricot yoghurt	200	13	20	low
Yoplait No Fat Banana Creamy Honey yoghurt	200	14	18	low
Yoplait No Fat Berry Brulée yoghurt	200	14	18	low
Yoplait No Fat Berry Crème yoghurt	200	14	16	low
Yoplait No Fat Black Cherry yoghurt	200	13	16	low
Yoplait No Fat Boysenberry yoghurt	200	12	16	low
Yoplait No Fat French Cheesecake yoghurt	200	14	18	low
Yoplait No Fat French Vanilla yoghurt	200	13	20	low
Yoplait No Fat Mango yoghurt	200	13	20	low
Yoplait No Fat Passionfruit Crème yoghurt	200	13	18	low
Yoplait No Fat Passionfruit yoghurt	200	13	20	low
Yoplait No Fat Peach Crème yoghurt	200	13	18	low
Yoplait No Fat Peach Mango yoghurt	200	13	20	low
Yoplait No Fat Raspberry yoghurt	200	13	16	low
Yoplait No Fat Strawberry yoghurt	200	12	16	low
Yoplait No Fat Tropical yoghurt	200	13	20	low

★ little or no carbs ■ high in saturated fat ⓖ GI Symbol partner

FOOD	NOMINAL SERVE SIZE g/ml	CARB (g)	GI	LOW MED HIGH
FAST FOOD & CONVENIENCE MEALS				
Sushi, salmon	100	36	48	low
Taco shells, cornmeal-based, baked	20	12	68	med

★ little or no carbs ■ high in saturated fat ⓒ GI Symbol partner

FOOD	NOMINAL SERVE SIZE g/ml	CARB (g)	GI	LOW MED HIGH
FRUIT				
Apple	120	15	38	low
Apple, dried	60	34	29	low
Apricots	168	13	57	med
Apricots, canned, in light syrup	120	19	64	med
Apricots, dried	60	28	30	low
Avocado	120	0	★	
Banana	120	26	52	low
Breadfruit	120	27	68	med
Cherries, dark	120	12	63	med
Cranberries, dried, sweetened	40	29	64	med
Custard apple	120	19	54	low
Dates, Arabic, vacuum-packed	55	41	39	low
Dates, pitted	60	40	45	high
Figs	50	4	★	
Figs, dried, tenderised, Dessert Maid	60	26	61	med
Fruit and nut mix	50	24	15	low
Fruit cocktail, canned	120	16	55	low
Grapefruit	120	11	25	low
Grapes	120	18	53	low
Kiwi fruit	120	12	53	low

★ little or no carbs ■ high in saturated fat ⓒ GI Symbol partner

FRUIT (CONT.)

FOOD	NOMINAL SERVE SIZE g/ml	CARB (g)	GI	LOW MED HIGH
Lemon	40	0	★	
Lime	40	0	★	
Lychees, canned, in syrup, drained	120	20	79	high
Mango	120	17	51	low
Mixed fruit, dried	60	41	60	med
Mixed nuts and raisins	50	16	21	low
Nectarine	120	9	43	low
Orange	120	11	42	low
Pawpaw	120	8	56	med
Peach	120	11	42	low
Peaches, canned, in heavy syrup	120	15	58	med
Peaches, canned, in light syrup	120	18	57	med
Peaches, canned, in natural juice	120	11	45	low
Peaches, dried	60	22	35	low
Pear	120	11	38	low
Pear, canned, in natural juice	120	13	44	low
Pear halves, canned, in reduced-sugar syrup, SPC Lite	120	14	25	low
Pears, dried	60	27	43	low
Pineapple	120	10	59	med

★ little or no carbs   ■ high in saturated fat   ⓖ GI Symbol partner

FOOD	NOMINAL SERVE SIZE g/ml	CARB (g)	GI	LOW MED HIGH
FRUIT (CONT.)				
Plum	120	12	39	low
Prunes, pitted, Sunsweet	60	33	29	low
Raisins	60	44	64	med
Raspberries	65	0	★	
Rhubarb	125	0	★	
Rockmelon	120	6	67	med
Strawberries	120	3	40	low
Sultanas	60	45	56	med
Tropical fruit and nut mix	50	28	49	low
Watermelon	120	6	76	high

★ little or no carbs   ■ high in saturated fat   © GI Symbol partner

FOOD	NOMINAL SERVE SIZE g/ml	CARB (g)	GI	LOW MED HIGH
GLUTEN-FREE PRODUCTS				
Buckwheat bread (Gluten and Wheat Free), Naturis Bakery	30	11	72	high
Buckwheat pancakes, gluten-free, packet mix, Orgran	77	22	102	high
Cookie, chocolate-coated, LEDA	30	14	35 ■	low
Corn pasta, Orgran	180	42	78	high
Corn Thins, Real Foods, puffed corn cakes, gluten-free	25	20	87	high
Muesli Breakfast Bar, gluten-free, Freedom Foods	35	20	50	low
Muesli (Gluten and Wheat Free with Psyllium), Freedom Foods	40	13	50	low
Muesli, with 1.5% fat milk, Freedom Foods	30	19	39	low
Multigrain bread, Country Life	30	13	79	high
Pancake Shake (Gluten, Wheat and Lactose free), Freedom Foods	80	53	61	med
Pasta, rice and maize, Ris'O'Mais, Orgran	180	49	76	high
Puffed Rice Cakes, white, Ricegrowers	25	21	82	high
Spaghetti, rice and split pea, canned in tomato sauce, Orgran	220	27	68	med

★ little or no carbs   ■ high in saturated fat   © GI Symbol partner

FOOD	NOMINAL SERVE SIZE g/ml	CARB (g)	GI	LOW MED HIGH
MEAT, SEAFOOD & PROTEIN				
Bacon	50	0	★■	
Beef, lean	120	0	★	
Brawn	75	0	★■	
Calamari rings, squid, not battered or crumbed	70	0	★	
Chicken, no skin	110	0	★	
Duck	140	0	★■	
Eggs	120	0	★■	
Fish	120	0	★	
Lamb	120	0	★	
Oysters, natural, plain	85	0	★	
Pork, lean	120	0	★	
Prawns	150	0	★	
Salmon, fresh or canned in water or brine	150	0	★	
Sardines	60	0	★	
Scallops, natural, plain	160	0	★	
Shellfish	120	0	★	
Steak, lean	120	0	★	
Tofu, bean curd, plain, unsweetened	100	0	★	
Trout, fresh or frozen	63	0	★	

★ little or no carbs ■ high in saturated fat ⓒ GI Symbol partner

FOOD	NOMINAL SERVE SIZE g/ml	CARB (g)	GI	LOW MED HIGH
MEAT, SEAFOOD & PROTEIN (CONT.)				
Tuna, fresh or canned in water or brine	120	0	★	
Turkey, lean	140	0	★	
Veal	120	0	★	

★ little or no carbs   ■ high in saturated fat   ⓒ GI Symbol partner

FOOD	NOMINAL SERVE SIZE g/ml	CARB (g)	GI	LOW MED HIGH
PASTA & NOODLES				
Corn pasta, gluten-free, boiled, Orgran®	180	46	68	med
Corn pasta, gluten-free, boiled, Orgran	180	42	78	high
Mung bean (Lungkow bean thread) noodles, dried, boiled	180	45	33	low
Noodles, dried rice, boiled	176	39	61	med
Noodles, fresh rice, boiled	180	39	40	low
Rice and maize pasta, Ris'O'Mais, gluten-free, Orgran	180	49	76	high
Rice pasta, brown, boiled	180	38	92	high
Rice vermicelli noodles, dried, boiled, Chinese	180	39	58	med
Soba noodles, instant, served in soup	180	49	46	low
Spaghetti, gluten-free, canned in tomato sauce, Orgran	220	27	68	med

★ little or no carbs   ■ high in saturated fat   ⓒ GI Symbol partner

FOOD	NOMINAL SERVE SIZE g/ml	CARB (g)	GI	LOW MED HIGH
RICE				
Arborio risotto rice, white, boiled, SunRice®	150	43	69	med
Basmati rice, white, boiled, Mahatma	150	38	58	med
Broken rice, Thai, white, cooked in rice cooker	150	43	86	high
Brown Pelde rice, boiled	150	38	76	high
Calrose rice, brown, medium-grain, boiled	150	40	87	high
Calrose rice, white, medium-grain, boiled	150	42	83	high
Doongara CleverRice™, SunRice, Ricegrowers	150	40	54	low
Doongara rice, white, boiled, Ricegrowers	150	39	56	med
Glutinous rice, white, cooked in rice cooker	150	32	98	high
Instant rice, white, cooked 6 mins with water	150	42	87	high
Jasmine fragrant rice, Sunrice, Ricegrowers	150	40	89	high
Jasmine rice, white, long-grain, cooked in rice cooker	150	42	109	high
Long-grain rice, white, Mahatma, boiled 15 mins	150	41	50	low
ⓖ Moolgiri rice	65	18	54	low
Pelde parboiled rice, Sungold	150	43	87	high
Sri Lankan Red Raw Rice	150	40	59	med

★ little or no carbs　■ high in saturated fat　ⓖ GI Symbol partner

FOOD	NOMINAL SERVE SIZE g/ml	CARB (g)	GI	LOW MED HIGH
RICE (CONT.)				
Sunbrown Quick® rice, Ricegrowers, boiled	150	38	80	high
SunRice Koshihikari rice, Ricegrowers	150	41	73	high
SunRice Medium Grain brown rice	125	43	59	med
SunRice Premium White Long Grain rice	150	40	59	med
Wild rice, boiled	164	32	57	med

★ little or no carbs ■ high in saturated fat ⓖ GI Symbol partner

THE GI GLUTEN-FREE TABLES **235**

FOOD	NOMINAL SERVE SIZE g/ml	CARB (g)	GI	LOW MED HIGH
SNACK FOODS				
Apricot and Yoghurt Healtheries Simple Bar, wheat and gluten free	50	25	40	low
Berry and Yoghurt Healtheries Simple Bar, wheat and gluten free	50	26	51	low
Cashew nuts, salted, Farmland	30	9	22	low
Chocolate, dark, plain, regular	30	19	41 ■	low
Chocolate Healtheries Simple bar, wheat and gluten free	50	27	35	low
Chocolate, milk, plain, Nestlé®	30	29	42 ■	low
Chocolate, milk, plain, reduced sugar	30	1	35 ■	low
Chocolate, milk, plain, regular	50	28	41 ■	low
Chocolate, milk, plain, with fructose instead of regular sugar	30	19	20 ■	low
Cookie, chocolate-coated, LEDA	30	14	35 ■	low
Corn chips, plain, salted	50	25	42 ■	low
Corn Thins, Real Foods, puffed corn cakes, gluten-free	25	20	87	high
Dove®, milk chocolate	48	29	45 ■	low
Jelly, diet, made from crystals with water	125	0	★	
Life Savers®, peppermint	30	30	70	high
Milky Bar®, white, Nestlé®	50	29	44 ■	low

★ little or no carbs   ■ high in saturated fat   ⓒ GI Symbol partner

FOOD	NOMINAL SERVE SIZE g/ml	CARB (g)	GI	LOW MED HIGH
SNACK FOODS				
Nuts, mixed, roasted and salted (dry roasted nuts may contain gluten)	50	17	24	low
Peanuts, roasted, salted (dry roasted nuts may contain gluten)	50	6	14	low
Pecan nuts, raw	50	3	10	low
Popcorn, plain, cooked in microwave	20	11	72	high
Potato chips, plain, salted (check for gluten)	50	18	54 ■	low
Roll-Ups®, processed fruit snack	30	25	99	high
Sesame seeds	11	0	★	
Snickers Bar®, regular	60	36	41 ■	low
ⓖ Sunripe School Straps Blackberry Sour Buzz	15	10	35	low
ⓖ Sunripe School Straps, dried fruit snack	15	11	40	low

★ little or no carbs   ■ high in saturated fat   ⓖ GI Symbol partner

FOOD	NOMINAL SERVE SIZE g/ml	CARB (g)	GI	LOW MED HIGH
SOY PRODUCTS				
Soy beans, canned, drained	150	6	14	low
Soy beans, dried, boiled	150	6	18	low
Vitasoy ® Lush, chocolate, reduced fat, soy milk	250	19	31	low
Vitasoy ® Lush, vanilla, reduced fat, soy milk	250	17	31	low
Vitasoy ® So Milky, regular, soy milk	250	8	21	low
Vitasoy ® So Milky, lite, soy milk	250	7	17	low

★ little or no carbs   ■ high in saturated fat   ⓖ GI Symbol partner

FOOD	NOMINAL SERVE SIZE g/ml	CARB (g)	GI	LOW MED HIGH
SPREADS & SWEETENERS				
Apricot fruit spread, reduced sugar, Glen Ewin	30	13	55	low
ⓖ Cottee's 100% Fruit Jam Apricot	15	9	50	low
ⓖ Cottee's 100% Fruit Jam Blackberry	15	9	46	low
ⓖ Cottee's 100% Fruit Jam Breakfast Marmalade	15	10	55	low
ⓖ Cottee's 100% Fruit Jam Raspberry	15	9	46	low
ⓖ Cottee's 100% Fruit Jam, Strawberry	15	9	46	low
Divine Date spread, Buderim Ginger	25	16	29	low
Fructose, pure	10	10	19	low
Ginger Marmalade, original, Buderim Ginger	18	13	50	low
Ginger spread, no cane sugar, Buderim Ginger	18	11	10	low
Ginger, sucrose-free, Buderim Ginger	20	15	10	low
Glucodin™ glucose tablets	10	10	100	high
Golden syrup	20	17	63	med
Grape jelly, Chateau Barrosa	15	10	52	low
Grape nectar, Chateau Barrosa	20	16	52	low
Grape syrup, Chateau Barrosa	15	16	52	low
Hommous, regular	30	5	6	low
Hommous, Chris' Traditional Hommous	30	5	22	low

★ little or no carbs ■ high in saturated fat ⓖ GI Symbol partner

FOOD	NOMINAL SERVE SIZE g/ml	CARB (g)	GI	LOW MED HIGH
SPREADS & SWEETENERS (CONT.)				
Honey, Capilano, blended	25	17	64	med
Honey, Ironbark	25	15	48	low
Honey, Red Gum	25	17	53	low
Honey, Salvation Jane	25	15	64	med
Honey, Stringybark	25	21	44	low
Honey, Yapunya	25	17	52	low
Honey, Yellowbox	25	18	35	low
Maple flavoured syrup, Cottee's®	25	22	68	med
Maple syrup, pure, Canadian	24	18	54	low
Marmalade, orange	30	20	55	low
Nutella®, hazelnut spread	20	12	33 ■	low
ⒼPremium Agave Nectar, Sweet Cactus Farms	5	3	19	low
Strawberry jam, regular	30	20	51	low
Sugar	10	10	60	med
ⒼSweetaddin	10	1	19	low
Vinegar (malt vinegar contains gluten)	5	0	★	

★ little or no carbs   ■ high in saturated fat   Ⓖ GI Symbol partner

FOOD	NOMINAL SERVE SIZE g/ml	CARB (g)	GI	LOW MED HIGH
VEGETABLES				
Alfalfa sprouts	6	0	★	
Artichokes, globe, fresh or canned in brine	80	0	★	
Asparagus	100	0	★	
Bean sprouts, raw	14	0	★	
Beetroot, canned	80	7	64	med
Bok choy	100	0	★	
Broccoli	60	0	★	
Brussels sprouts	100	0	★	
Cabbage	70	0	★	
Capsicum	80	0	★	
Carrots, peeled, boiled	80	5	41	low
Cauliflower	60	0	★	
Celery	40	0	★	
Chillies, fresh or dried	20	0	★	
Chives, fresh	4	0	★	
Cucumber	45	0	★	
Eggplant	100	0	★	
Endive	30	0	★	
Fennel	90	0	★	
Garlic	5	0	★	

★ little or no carbs ■ high in saturated fat © GI Symbol partner

FOOD	NOMINAL SERVE SIZE g/ml	CARB (g)	GI	LOW MED HIGH
VEGETABLES (CONT.)				
Ginger	10	0	★	
Herbs, fresh or dried	2	0	★	
Kumara, boiled	150	21	77	high
Leeks	80	0	★	
Lettuce	50	0	★	
Mushrooms	35	0	★	
Okra	80	0	★	
Onions, raw, peeled	30	0	★	
Parsnips	80	8	52	low
Potatoes, Almera, boiled	150	15	65	med
Potatoes, Carisma, boiled	150	20	55	low
Potatoes, Desiree, peeled, boiled 35 mins	150	17	101	high
Potatoes, Nardine, peeled, boiled	150	25	70	high
Potatoes, new, canned, microwaved 3 mins	150	18	65	med
Potatoes, Nicola, unpeeled, boiled whole 15 minutes	150	16	58	med
Potatoes, Pontiac, peeled, boiled 15 mins, mashed	150	20	91	high
Potatoes, Pontiac, peeled, boiled whole 30–35 mins	150	18	72	high
Potatoes, Pontiac, peeled, microwaved 7 mins	150	18	79	high

★ little or no carbs ■ high in saturated fat Ⓖ GI Symbol partner

VEGETABLES (CONT.)

FOOD	NOMINAL SERVE SIZE g/ml	CARB (g)	GI	LOW MED HIGH
Potatoes, Sebago, peeled, boiled 35 mins	150	17	87	high
Pumpkin, Butternut	80	6	51	low
Radishes	15	0	★	
Rocket	30	0	★	
Shallots	10	0	★	
Silverbeet	35	0	★	
Snow pea sprouts	15	0	★	
Spinach	75	0	★	
Spring onions	15	0	★	
Squash, yellow	70	0	★	
Swede, cooked	150	10	72	high
Sweet corn, honey and pearl variety, boiled (New Zealand)	150	30	37	low
Sweet corn, on the cob, boiled	80	16	48	low
Sweet corn, whole kernel, canned, drained	80	14	46	low
Sweet potato, purple skin, white flesh (Australia)	150	30	75	high
Sweet potato, orange flesh, boiled (Australia)	150	18	61	med
Taro	150	8	54	low
Tomato	150	0	★	

★ little or no carbs ■ high in saturated fat © GI Symbol partner

FOOD	NOMINAL SERVE SIZE g/ml	CARB (g)	GI	LOW MED HIGH
VEGETABLES (CONT.)				
Turnip	120	0	★	
Watercress	8	0	★	
Yam, peeled, boiled	150	36	37	low
Zucchini	100	0	★	

★ little or no carbs ■ high in saturated fat ⊙ GI Symbol partner

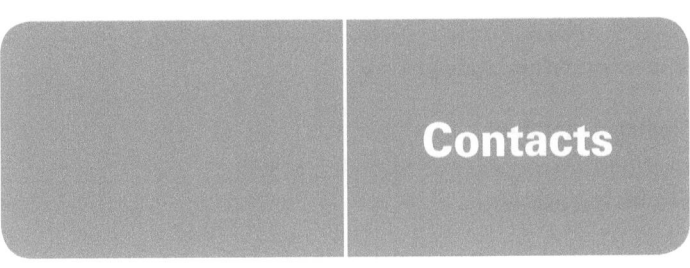

Contacts

For further information on GI

www.glycemicindex.com
This is the University of Sydney's glycemic index website where you can learn about GI and access the GI database which includes the most up-to-date listing of the GI of foods that have been published in international scientific journals.

www.gisymbol.com.au
The Glycemic Index (GI) Symbol Program is a food labelling program with strict nutritional criteria that aims to help people make informed food choices. The site includes a complete listing of foods carrying the GI symbol.

http://ginews.blogspot.com
GI News is the University of Sydney Human Nutrition Unit's official glycemic index monthly newsletter. Subscribing is free.

FOR INFORMATION ON:

Food labelling and food additives
Food Standards Australia New Zealand (FSANZ)
www.foodstandards.gov.au

Finding a dietitian
Dietitians Association of Australia (DAA)
www.daa.asn.au

New Zealand Dietetic Association (NZDA)
www.dietitians.org.nz

Diabetes
Diabetes Australia
www.diabetesaustralia.com.au

Diabetes New Zealand
www.diabetes.org.nz

Heart health
National Heart Foundation Australia
www.heartfoundation.org.au

National Heart Foundation of New Zealand
www.heartfoundation.org.nz

Te Hotu Manawa Maori
This is a national health promotion organisation with the specific aim of reducing the likelihood of heart-related illness and death amongst Maori. They undertake training courses for Maori in nutrition and physical activity.
www.tehotumanawa.org.nz

Coeliac Disease
Coeliac Australia
www.coeliac.org.au

Coeliac New Zealand
www.coeliac.org.nz

Other helpful websites and specialist online stores

www.coeliac.com.au
The Sue Shepherd website provides information about coeliac disease, fructose and IBS resources.

www.glutenfreeshop.com.au
This website allows users to filter products by intolerance before ordering gluten-free foods for home delivery.

www.glutenfreegoodies.co.nz
The Gluten Free Goodies Company offers dry, gluten-free ingredient mixes, baking powder and recipes.

www.celiac.ca
The Canadian Celiac Association is a national organisation dedicated to providing services and support to persons with celiac disease and dermatitis herpetiformis through programs of awareness, advocacy, education and research.

www.coeliac.org.uk
Coeliac UK is the only national charity supporting people with coeliac disease in the UK. It is also the biggest coeliac society in the world and regularly shares knowledge and advice with international colleagues.

www.csaceliacs.org
The Celiac Sprue Association (CSA) is a worldwide member-based nonprofit organisation which aims to increase awareness, improve diagnosis and treatment, and help all coeliacs worldwide manage the gluten-free lifestyle. The CSA vision is 'Celiacs Helping Celiacs'.

www.celiac.com/glutenfreemall
Online special diet superstore, The Gluten-Free Mall® was created by Scott Adams, better known in the coeliac/gluten-free community for founding Celiac.com. Features a selection of gluten-free, wheat-free, casein-free and other allergy-related health foods and special dietary products on the Internet. All featured products are specifically designed for people who need to be on a gluten-free diet due to coeliac disease, autism, Attention Deficit Hyperactivity Disorder (ADD, ADHD) or other health reasons.

www.glutenfreeliving.com
A US magazine, *Gluten-Free Living* provides practical, reliable information about the gluten-free diet, and is known for extensive and reliable research into ingredients and the gluten-free diet. The editors use their journalism experience to investigate and clear-up misinformation about the gluten-free diet.

www.GFlinks.com
On the web since 1996, the Gluten-Free Page with good listings of links specific to coeliac disease/gluten intolerance websites. Features: popular sites, books, educational institutions, journals, coeliac associations and commercial sites.

www.herbies.com.au
Herbie's spices are gluten-free, except for asafoetida and blends containing asafoetida.

Acknowledgements

Despite the digital age, publishing a book isn't one of those things that magically happens. There's a big team in the background researching, checking, commenting, designing.

So, first we would like to thank Fiona Hazard and Bernadette Foley at Hachette Australia who signed us up to write the book, our original publisher Vanessa Radnidge, and production editor Anna Waddington. Thank you for listening to our ideas and bringing the book to life. We also greatly appreciate the efforts of our editors Jacquie Brown and Julia Nekich; proofreader Pamela Dunne; and designer Judi Rowe. Special thanks to Helen Littleton, our new publisher; and Kate Ballard, our editor, for their assistance and patience in updating and revising this edition.

Diane Temple has played an absolutely key role in helping us put this book together. We simply could not have done it without her. Diane has been wonderful to work with developing and testing the recipes to meet our nutritional guidelines. Nothing was ever too much to ask – even using legumes in baking cakes! And we are also grateful to her intrepid taste test team: daughter Ava and husband Ben Gerstel.

We would like to thank Sydney University Glycemic Index Research Manager Fiona Atkinson for sharing her work and providing us with the latest GI values right up to the last minute; and Alan Barclay for giving us a template to work from as we compiled the tables.

We would also like to thank Sue Shepherd for writing the foreword and the team at Coeliac Australia for their support and endorsement.

Last, we thank our families for their encouragement and support – Lee Dixon (Kate's mum, who made lots of great suggestions), John Miller and Roger Sandall.

About the authors

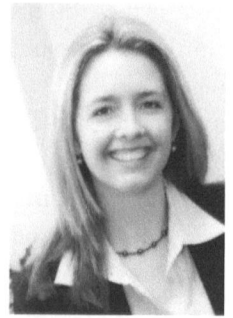

Dr Kate Marsh is an Advanced Accredited Practicing Dietitian and Credentialled Diabetes Educator, with a Masters of Nutrition and Dietetics from the University of Sydney and a Graduate Certificate in Diabetes Education and Management from the University of Technology, Sydney. She has also completed her PhD at the University of Sydney looking at the benefits of a low GI diet for women with PCOS.

Kate works in private practice in Sydney and has a particular interest in diabetes, insulin resistance, polycystic ovary syndrome (PCOS), coeliac disease and vegetarian nutrition. She currently chairs the DAA National PCOS and the Vegetarian Interest Groups and is co-chair of the DAA National Diabetes Interest Group.

Kate writes regularly for a number of publications including *Diabetic Living*, *Healthy Food Guide*, *Nature & Health* and *Orgran's Everyday Health Magazine* and is co-author of *The Low GI Diet for Polycystic Ovarian Syndrome* and *The Low GI Vegetarian Cookbook*. She was the 2006 recipient of the DAA Young Achievers Award, a NSW finalist in the 2006 Telstra Business Women's Awards and in 2010 received the Joan Woodhill Prize for Excellence in Research – Doctorate Award for her PhD study in women with PCOS.

ABOUT THE AUTHORS

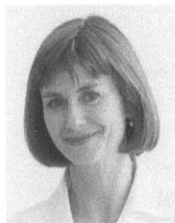

Professor Jennie-Brand Miller is Professor of Human Nutrition at the University of Sydney, immediate past Chair of the National Nutrition Committee of the Australian Academy of Science, a past President of the Nutrition Society of Australia, the Director of Sydney University Glycemic Index Research Services (SUGiRS, a GI testing service for the food industry) and President of the non-profit Glycemic Index Foundation, which administers a food symbol program for consumers in collaboration with Diabetes Australia and the Juvenile Diabetes Research Foundation.

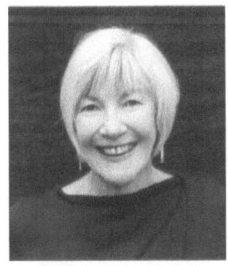

Philippa Sandall is the Editor of GI News (http://ginews.blogspot.com), the official online newsletter published by the University of Sydney's GI Group. As a keen cook, writer and editor, she specialises in food, health and nutrition and has played a leading role in developing and publishing the *Low GI Diet* series worldwide since 1995. Her most recent book is *Money Saving Meals* (with Diane Temple).

Index

7-day menus
  adult, 78–79
  adult vegetarian, 80–81
  schoolchild, 84–85
  teenager, 82–83

A

abdominal fat, 27
Accredited Practising Dietitian (APD), 12, 13
adult 7-day menu, 78–79
adult vegetarian 7-day menu, 80–81
age, 8
alcohol, 72
alfalfa, 240
allergies, food, 13
amylose, 41
apple, 226
apricots, 226
arborio rice, 42, 233
artichokes, 240
asparagus, 240
autism, 13
avocados, 226

B

bacon, 230
baked beans, 205
bananas, 226
beans, 205–206
bean sprouts, 240
beetroot, 240
beverages, 71–72
  GI gluten-free tables, 207–209
biscuits, 73, 210, 229
blood glucose levels
  GI (glycemic index) and, 23–25
  GL (glycemic load) and, 44
  high, 27
  in pregnancy, 34
  starch digestion and, 25–26, 28
bok choy, 240
brawn, 230
bread
  GI gluten-free tables, 211, 229
  GI value of, 39
  low GI gluten-free baking, 74
  low GI varieties, 73
  serving size, 52
breadfruit, 226
breakfast. *see also* 7-day menus
  breads and cereals, 53
  fish and seafood, 67
  fruits and vegetables, 50
  lean meats and dairy, 63
  legumes, 56
  nuts and seeds, 60
breakfast bars, 229
breakfast cereals, 53, 73
  GI gluten-free tables, 212–213
  GI value of, 39–40
broccoli, 240
brown rice, 41–42, 233
brussels sprouts, 240

C

cabbage, 240
cakes, 73, 214
calcium, 61
canola oil, 69
capsicum, 240
carbohydrates. *see also* high GI carbohydrates; low GI carbohydrates; starches; sugars
  conversion of, 28
  GI (glycemic index) of, 23–24
  GL (glycemic load) and, 44
  simple *versus* complex, 24
carrots, 240
casein-free diet, 13
cauliflower, 240
celery, 240
cereals. *see* breakfast cereals; whole cereal grains
cheese, 43–44, 61, 216
cherries, 226
chestnuts, 43
chicken, 62, 70, 71, 230
chickpeas, 205
children
  infant birth weights, 34

obesity in, 34
schoolchild 7-day menu, 84–85
chillies, 240
chocolate, 235
chocolate drinks, 208
chocolate milk, 219, 235
cholesterol, 61–62
Coeliac Australia, 246
coeliac disease, 7–9
  symptoms of, 9–10
Coeliac New Zealand, 247
coffee, 72, 207
coffee milk, 219
condensed milk, 219
convenience meals, 74–75, 225
cookies, 229, 235
cordial, 207
crackers, 73, 210, 229
cranberries, 226
crispbreads, 73, 210, 229
cucumber, 240
custards, 216–218
custard apple, 226

D

dairy foods. *see also* cheese; milk; yoghurt
  GI gluten-free tables, 216–218
  GI value of, 43
  in gluten-free diet, 61–65
  saturated products, 71
  serving size, 63
dates, 226
dermatitis herpetiformis, 7, 10–11
  symptoms of, 11
desserts. *see* snacks and desserts
DH. *see* dermatitis herpetiformis
diabetes
  gestational, 27, 34
  type 1, 27, 29–30, 34
  type 2, 26, 27, 29–30
Diabetes Australia, 246
Diabetes New Zealand, 246
Dietitians Association of Australia, 246
digestion of starch, 25–26, 28
dinner. *see also* 7-day menus
  breads and cereals, 53
  fish and seafood, 67–68
  fruits and vegetables, 51
  lean meats and dairy, 64
  legumes, 56
  nuts and seeds, 60
dips, 238
drinks, 71–72
  GI gluten-free tables, 207–209
duck, 230

E

eating out, 74–75, 225
eggplant, 240
eggs
  GI gluten-free tables, 230
  in gluten-free diet, 61–62
  monounsaturated fat in, 70
elimination diet, 12, 13
endive, 240
energy water, 209

F

familial hypercholesterol-emia, 62
fast food, 74–75, 225
fat as macronutrient, 65. *see also* oils and fats
fatty liver disease, 27
fennel, 240
fibre, 20–21, 89
figs, 226
fish
  GI gluten-free tables, 230–231
  in gluten-free diet, 66–68
  polyunsaturated products, 70
  serving size, 67
flaxseed oil, 69–70
flours, 74, 88, 92
fluids, 71–72
  GI gluten-free tables, 207–209
foods. *see also* low GI carbohydrates
  sources of insoluble fibre, 21
  sources of soluble fibre, 20
  suitable for gluten-free diet, 16–17
  unsuitable for gluten-free diet, 17–18

food additives, 246
food allergies, 13
food labels, 19, 245, 246
Foods Standards Code, 19
free radicals, 30
fruits
    GI gluten-free tables, 226–228
    GI value of, 37–38
    in gluten-free diet, 48–51
    serving size, 48–49
fruit and nut mix, 226
fruit juice, 71–72, 207–208
fruit, mixed, 227

G
garlic, 240
genetic testing, 10
gestational diabetes, 27, 34
GI (glycemic index)
    of carbohydrates, 23–24
    database of GI values, 204
    diabetes and, 29–30
    digestion of starch, 25–26, 28
    heart disease and, 30–31
    PCOS and, 33
    pregnancy and, 34
ginger, 241
GL (glycemic load), 44
glucose, 28, 53
gluten, 7, 8
gluten-free diet
    autism and, 13
    benefits of low GI carbohydrates in, 21, 24
    foods suitable for, 16–17
    foods unsuitable for, 17–18
    GI tables for, 201–204
gluten-free food websites, 16
'gluten-free' label, 19
Gluten-Free Living, 248
gluten intolerance, 7, 11–12
glycemic index. *see* GI
Glycemic Index (GI) Symbol Program, 245
glycemic load (GL), 44
glycogen, 28
grains. *see* whole cereal grains
grapefruit, 226
grapes, 226
green tea, 72

H
heart disease, 30–31, 246
herbs, 240, 241
herbal teas, 72
heredity, 7–8
high GI carbohydrates
    breakdown of, 23, 25
    combined with low GI carbohydrates, 26
    low GI substitutes for, 73
    weight loss and, 31–32
honey, 239
hormones, stress, 32
hunger, 32–33

I
ice-cream, 216–218
immune reactions, 8
immunoglobulin A (IgA), 11
impaired glucose tolerance, 27
insoluble fibre, 20–21
insulin
    in conversion of carbohydrates, 28
    levels of, 26–27
    resistance to, 29, 33, 35
insulin resistance syndrome, 27
iron, 61
irritable bowel syndrome, 12

J
jams, 238–239

K
kilojoules, 89
kiwi fruit, 226

L
labels. *see* food labels
lactose intolerance, 61
lean meats
    alternatives to, 61
    GI gluten-free tables, 230–231
    in gluten-free diet, 61–64
    monounsaturated products, 70

no GI values, 65
saturated products, 71
serving size, 62
leeks, 241
legumes
as alternatives to meat, 61
dried and canned, 58
GI gluten-free tables, 205–206
GI value of, 42–43
in gluten-free diet, 54–58
serving size, 56
lemons, 227
lentils, 206
lettuce, 241
limes, 227
linseed oil, 69–70
liver, 61–62
low GI carbohydrates
benefits for gluten-free diet, 21, 24
combined with high GI carbohydrates, 26
medical conditions helped by, 27
substitutes for high GI carbohydrates, 73
weight loss and, 32–33
'low gluten' label, 19
lunch. *see also* 7-day menus
breads and cereals, 53
fish and seafood, 67
fruits and vegetables, 50–51
lean meats and dairy, 63–64
legumes, 56
nuts and seeds, 60
lychees, 227

M

mangoes, 227
maple syrup, 239
margarine, 92
meats. *see* lean meats
metabolic syndrome, 27
milk
flavoured, 207, 219
GI gluten-free tables, 219–220
GI value of, 72
in gluten-free diet, 61
minerals, 61
mineral water, 71

monounsaturated products, 70
muesli bars, 229
muffins, 73, 214
mung beans, 206
mushrooms, 241

N

NAFLD, 27
NASH, 27
nectarines, 227
New Zealand Dietetic Association, 246
non-coeliac gluten sensitivity, 7, 11–12
noodles
GI gluten-free tables, 232
GI value of, 40–41
glucose and, 53
low GI varieties, 73
nuts and seeds
GI gluten-free tables, 235–236
GI value of, 43
in gluten-free diet, 58–60
low GI varieties, 73
monounsaturated products, 70
polyunsaturated products, 70
serving size, 59

O

oats, 7, 42, 213
oils and fats
no GI values, 65
omega-3 fats, 62, 66, 68–69
omega-6 fats, 68–69
polyunsaturated and monounsaturated, 70
saturated, 61, 71, 89
okra, 241
olive oil, 69
omega-3 fats, 62, 66, 68–69
omega-6 fats, 68–69
onions, 241
oranges, 227
overweight, 27, 34

P

pancakes, 229
pancreas, 29

parsnips, 241
pasta
  GI gluten-free tables, 229, 232
  GI value of, 40–41, 92
  glucose and, 53
  low GI varieties, 73
pawpaw, 227
PCOS (polycystic ovarian syndrome), 27, 33
peaches, 227
peanut oil, 69
pears, 227
peas, 206
pineapple, 227
plums, 228
polyunsaturated products, 70
popcorn, 236
porridge, 73, 213
potatoes
  GI gluten-free tables, 241–242
  GI value of, 38
  low GI varieties, 73, 92–93
  serving size, 49
pre-diabetes, 27
pregnancy, 34
processed foods, 26
processed meats, 71
protein
  alternatives to meats, 61
  GI gluten-free tables, 230–231
  importance of, 90
  no GI values, 65
prunes, 228
pulses. *see* legumes
pumpkin, 242

R
radishes, 242
raisins, 228
raspberries, 228
red meat. *see* lean meats
rhubarb, 228
rice
  GI gluten-free tables, 233–234
  GI value of, 41–42
  glucose and, 53
  low GI varieties, 73, 93

rice desserts, 217–218
rocket, 242
rockmelon, 228

S
salt, 88
saturated products, 71
seafood
  GI gluten-free tables, 230–231
  in gluten-free diet, 66–68
  serving size, 67
seeds. *see* nuts and seeds
shallots, 93, 242
silverbeet, 242
snacks and desserts
  breads and cereals, 53
  dairy, 65
  fruits and vegetables, 51
  GI gluten-free tables, 216–218, 235–236
  legumes, 56
  nuts and seeds, 60
snow pea sprouts, 242
soda water, 71
sodium, 88
soft drinks, 207–208
soluble fibre, 20–21
soy beans, 206, 237
soy bean curd, 55, 61, 230
soy products
  GI gluten-free tables, 220, 237
  GI value of, 43, 72
  in gluten-free diet, 61
  polyunsaturated products, 70
spices, 93
spinach, 242
split peas, 206
spreads, 70, 71, 92
  GI gluten-free tables, 238–239
spring onions, 93, 242
squash, 242
starches
  digestion of, 25–26, 28
  GI and, 24–25
stock, 93
strawberries, 228
stress hormones, 32

sugars
  GI and, 24–25
  GI gluten-free tables, 239
sultanas, 228
sushi, 225
swede, 242
sweet potato, 49, 73, 241, 242
sweetcorn, 49, 73, 242
sweeteners, 238–239
symptoms
  of coeliac disease, 9–10
  of dermatitis herpetiformis, 11
syndrome X, 27

T
taco, 225
tamari, 93
taro, 242
Te Hotu Manawa Maori, 246
teas, 72
teenager 7-day menu, 82–83
tofu, 55, 61, 230
tomato, 242
triglyceride levels, 27
turkey, 231
turnip, 243
type 1 diabetes, 27, 29–30, 34
type 2 diabetes, 26, 27, 29–30

V
vegetables
  GI gluten-free tables, 240–243
  GI value of, 38
  in gluten-free diet, 48–51
  serving size, 49
  starchy, 49–50
vegetable juice, 207–209
villous atrophy, 10, 11

vinegar, 239
vitamins, 61

W
water, 71
watercress, 243
watermelon, 228
websites
  GI, 245
  for gluten-free foods, 16
  specialist online stores, 247–248
weight
  childhood obesity, 34
  overweight, 27, 34
  weight control, 31, 90
  weight loss, 31–32
wheat allergy, 13
wheat-free breakfast cereals, 213
wheat intolerance, 12–13
whole cereal grains
  GI gluten-free tables, 215
  GI value of, 41–42
  in gluten-free diet, 52–54
  serving size, 52
wild rice, 42, 234

X
xanthan gum, 94

Y
yam, 243
yoghurt
  GI gluten-free tables, 221–225
  in gluten-free diet, 61

Z
zinc, 61
zucchini, 243

Index of recipes

almonds
  chocolate almond cake 188
  granola with 98
  orange almond dessert cake 192
apples
  apple and pecan muffins 112
  cranberry baked apples 189
  multigrain porridge with apple 104
  pork with glazed apple and cannellini mash 172
  rhubarb and apple crumble 191
apricot
  apricot and strawberry parfait crunch 102
  apricot nut slice 121
avocado
  carrot, avocado and snow pea rice paper rolls 135
  tofu hotcakes with avocado, tomato and corn salsa 108
  turkey, avocado and fresh peach salsa wraps 106

baking tips 117
bananas 99
  banana and passionfruit smoothie 99
  banana walnut loaf 115
  passionfruit banana cups 186
  ricotta, strawberry and banana wraps 105
beans
  beef and bean fajitas 124
  butter bean salad 132
  cannellini mash 172
  fennel, bean and tomato salad 161
  Mexican black bean soup with corn 155
beef
  beef and bean fajitas 124
  Greek-style beef skewers 169
  Thai beef salad with chilli lime dressing 142

berries 101
  berry and pear cobbler 182
  berry yoghurt delight 183
  muesli with 97
biscuits, muesli nut 119
bok choy, pork and noodle stir-fry 174
breakfasts 97–110
  basics 195
  breakfast fried rice 107
brownies 118
brunches 97–110

cakes
  chocolate almond 188
  orange almond dessert cake 192
cannellini mash 172
  potato and 197
carrot
  carrot, avocado and snow pea rice paper rolls 135
  corn, carrot and onion muffins 114
casserole, fruity lamb 168
cereal 95
cherry chocolate muffins 113
chicken
  barbecued lemon chicken skewers 162
  chicken and corn soup 158
  chicken and rice lettuce cups 145
  chicken mango rice paper rolls 134
  chicken nuggets with salad 125
  chicken pasta salad with mango salsa 144
  chicken tacos 126
  cranberry chicken with quinoa 164
  poaching 196
  stock 196
chickpeas, tomato soup with 157
chilli
  chilli lime dressing 142
  chipotle chilli in adobo sauce 198
chipotle chilli in adobo sauce 198

chocolate
   cherry chocolate muffins 113
   chocolate almond cake 188
   chocolate mousse 185
   no-bake chocolate clusters 120
cobbler, berry and pear 182
coconut and lime macaroons 187
corn
   chicken and corn soup 158
   corn and coriander fritters 128
   corn, carrot and onion muffins 114
   Mexican black bean soup with corn 155
   tofu hotcakes with avocado, tomato and corn salsa 108
cranberries
   cranberry baked apples 189
   cranberry chicken with quinoa 164
curries
   lamb curry with spinach rice pilaf 170
   Madras curry blend 199
custard apple and orange smoothie 100

desserts 181–94
dressings
   chilli lime 142

fajitas, beef and bean 124
falafel wraps 127
feta and lentil salad 150
fish
   herb fish parcels with fennel, bean and tomato salad 161
fried rice, breakfast 107
fritters, corn and coriander 107
fruit loaf 116

granola with pecans and almonds 98
Greek-style beef skewers 169
guacamole 197
herb blend, Italian 199
herb fish parcels with fennel, bean and tomato salad 161
hommous 196

Italian herb blend 199
Italian meatballs in tomato sauce 131
Italian rice and lentil soup 153

jelly, yoghurt strawberry 194

laksa, prawn 154
lamb
   fruity lamb casserole 168
   lamb curry with spinach rice pilaf 170
lasagne, pumpkin, ricotta and lentil 176
legumes, tips for 193
lemon
   barbecued lemon chicken skewers 162
   lemon delicious pudding 190
lentils
   Italian rice and lentil soup 153
   lentil and feta salad 150
   lentil mash 197
   pumpkin, ricotta and lentil lasagne 176
light meals 123–39
lime and coconut macaroons 187
loaves
   banana walnut loaf 115
   fruit loaf 116
lunchbox tips 137
lunches 123–29

macaroons, coconut and lime 187
Madras curry blend 199
mains 159–80
mango
   chicken mango rice paper rolls 134
   chicken pasta salad with mango salsa 144
meatballs, Italian, in tomato sauce 131
meringues 184
Mexican black bean soup with corn 155

Moroccan seafood stew 180
mousse, chocolate 185
muesli
  berries, with 97
  muesli nut biscuits 119
muffins
  apple and pecan 112
  cherry chocolate 113
  corn, carrot and onion 114
multigrain porridge with apple 104

no-bake chocolate clusters 120
noodles
  gluten-free 175
  pork, bok choy and noodle stir-fry 174

onion
  corn, carrot and onion muffins 114
orange
  orange almond dessert cake 192
  orange and custard apple smoothie 100

pad Thai, vegetarian 178
passionfruit and banana smoothie 99
passionfruit banana cups 186
pasta
  chicken pasta salad with mango salsa 144
  pasta salads 149
  tuna pasta nicoise 148
patties, salmon and pumpkin, with butter bean salad 132
peaches
  peachy pistachio porridge 103
  turkey, avocado and fresh peach salsa wraps 106
pear and berry cobbler 182
pecans
  apple and pecan muffins 112
  granola with pecans and almonds 98
pistachios
  peachy pistachio porridge 103
  pistachio and quinoa tabbouli 147

pizza
  portobello pizzas with parmesan crumb 110
pork
  glazed apple and cannellini mash, with 172
  pork, bok choy and noodle stir-fry 174
porridge
  multigrain, with apple 104
  peachy pistachio 103
portobello pizzas with parmesan crumb 110
potatoes
  potato and cannellini mash 197
  sweet potato mash 198
  warm potato salad with herbs and toasted hazelnuts 143
prawn laksa 154
pudding, lemon delicious 190
pumpkin
  pumpkin, ricotta and lentil lasagne 176
  pumpkin soup 152
  salmon and pumpkin patties with butter bean salad 132

quinoa
  cranberry chicken with 164
  quick and easy 165
  quinoa and pistachio tabbouli 147

rhubarb and apple crumble 191
rice
  breakfast fried rice 107
  brown 146
  chicken and rice lettuce cups 145
  Italian rice and lentil soup 153
  lamb curry with spinach rice pilaf 170
  wild 146
rice paper rolls
  carrot, avocado and snow pea 135
  chicken mango 134
  tuna 136
ricotta
  pumpkin, ricotta and lentil lasagne 176

INDEX OF RECIPES

ricotta, strawberry and banana wraps 105

salads 141–58
  butter bean 132
  chicken nuggets with 125
  chicken pasta salad with mango salsa 144
  fennel, bean and tomato salad 161
  lentil and feta salad 150
  pasta salads 149
  Thai beef salad with chilli lime dressing 142
  warm potato salad with herbs and toasted hazelnuts 143
salmon and pumpkin patties with butter bean salad 132
salsa
  avocado, tomato and corn salsa 108
  fresh peach 106
  mango 144
seafood stew, Moroccan 180
skewers
  barbecued lemon chicken skewers 162
  Greek-style beef 169
slice, apricot nut 121
smoothies
  banana and passionfruit 99
  custard apple and orange 100
  strawberry 101
snacks 111–22
snow peas
  carrot, avocado and snow pea rice paper rolls 135
soups 141–58
  chicken and corn soup 158
  Italian rice and lentil 153
  Mexican black bean soup with corn 155
  pumpkin 152
  tomato soup with chickpeas 157
Spanish tortillas 130
spice blends 199

spinach
  lamb curry with spinach rice pilaf 170
stew, Moroccan seafood 180
stir-fries
  pork, bok choy and noodle stir-fry 174
strawberries
  apricot and strawberry parfait crunch 102
  ricotta, strawberry and banana wraps 105
  strawberry sauce 200
  strawberry smoothie 101
  yoghurt strawberry jelly 194
sushi with three fillings 138
sweet potato mash 198

tabbouli, pistachio and quinoa 147
tacos, chicken 126
Thai beef salad with chilli lime dressing 142
toast 95
  toast-topper tips 109
tofu hotcakes with avocado, tomato and corn salsa 108
tomato
  fennel, bean and tomato salad 161
  tofu hotcakes with avocado, tomato and corn salsa 108
  tomato soup with chickpeas 157
tomato sauce, Italian meatballs in 131
tortillas, Spanish 130
treats 111–22
tuna
  tuna bake 166
  tuna pasta nicoise 148
  tuna rice paper rolls 136
turkey, avocado and fresh peach salsa wraps 106

vegetarian pad Thai 178

walnuts
  banana walnut loaf 115

wraps
    falafel wraps 127
    ricotta, strawberry and banana 105
    turkey, avocado and fresh peach salsa wraps 106

yoghurt
    berry yoghurt delight 183
    yoghurt strawberry jelly 194

PROFESSOR JENNIE BRAND-MILLER'S
Low GI DIET Cookbooks

Delicious and healthy GI-friendly recipes from the low-GI eating pioneers.

The Low GI Vegetarian Cookbook
A collection of over eighty delicious and tempting recipes, illustrated with mouth-watering photography including recipes for breakfasts, light lunches and snacks, main courses and desserts and sweet treats including Asian, Indian and Mediterranean style dishes.

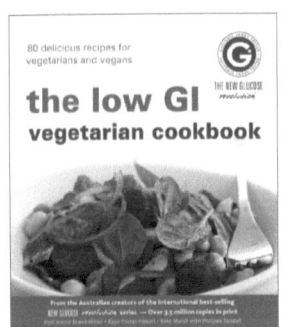

The Low GI Family Cookbook
Whether you have a toddler or a teenager, this cookbook shows you how easy it is to combine the essentials of healthy eating with the proven benefits of low GI carbs and make a real difference to your whole family's long-term health and wellbeing – with over 100 healthy recipes the whole family will love.

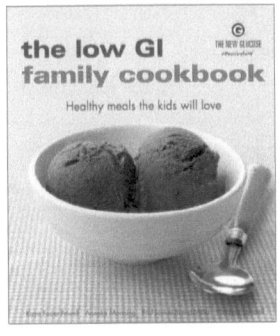

The Low GI Diet Cookbook
Science has proven that low GI, slowly digested carbohydrates are key to healthy and sustained weight loss. *The Low GI Diet Cookbook* brings you over seventy tempting recipes based on these established principles. Packed with beautiful photographs, handy tips, and with a complete breakdown of fat, protein and carb content, calorie values and GI values for every recipe, covering everything from sustaining breakfasts and brunches, substantial but healthy dinner dishes, to quick salads and sweet treats.

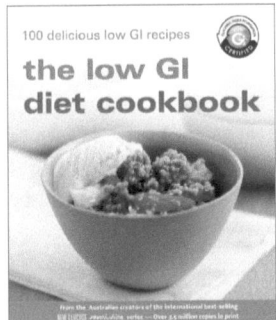

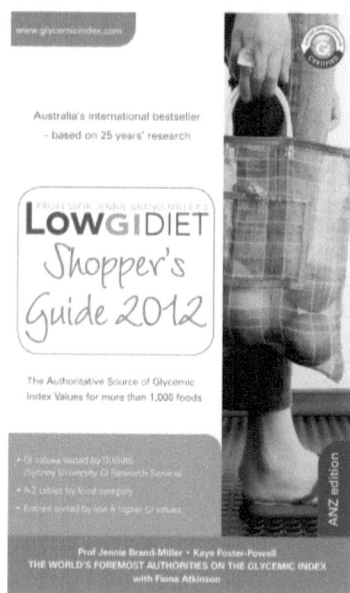

Find all the latest GI values with Australia's #1 low GI shopper's guide.

GI values are the key to lowering the GI of your diet. This guide will help you compare your favourite foods and preferred brands so you can make the substitutions that really matter. In this easy-to-use book we give you:

- **The GI values of over 1,000 foods**
- **A–Z tables by food category**
- **A low or high GI rating for each food**
- **Handy household measures and expanded nutrient data for each food – carbohydrate content and glycemic load per serving**
- **A shopping list of low GI essentials**
- **A guide to eating out**
- **Healthy takeaway food options**
- **Ideas for gluten-free eating and living**
- **Sugars and sweeteners section**

www.ingramcontent.com/pod-product-compliance
Ingram Content Group UK Ltd.
Pitfield, Milton Keynes, MK11 3LW, UK
UKHW041229200426
11947UKWH00035B/581